PCCN Study Guide
2024-2025

Review Book with 375 Practice Questions and Answer Explanations for the Progressive Care Certified Nurse Exam

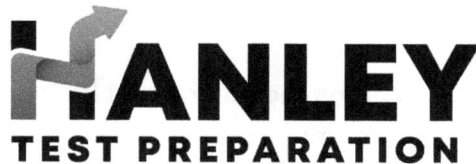

HANLEY
TEST PREPARATION

Contents

Free Video Offer!

Thank you for purchasing from Hanley Test Preparation! We're honored to help you prepare for your exam. To show our appreciation, we're offering an Exclusive Test Tips Video.

This video includes multiple strategies that will make you successful on your big exam.

All we ask is that you email us your feedback and describe your experience with our product. Amazing, awful, or just so-so. We want to hear what you have to say!

To get your FREE VIDEO, just send us an email at bonusvideo@hanleytestprep.com with **Free Video** in the subject line and the following information in the body of the email:

- The name of the product you purchased
- Your product rating on a scale of 1-5, with 5 being the highest rating.
- Your feedback about the product.

If you have any questions or concerns, please don't hesitate to contact us at support@hanleytestprep.com

Thanks again!

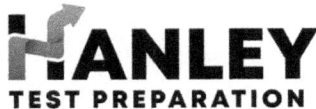

TEST PREPARATION

Introduction

The nursing profession has come a long way since Florence Nightingale's time. It is one of the most lucrative and challenging professions for women who want to balance home and career. Let's review the current data on nursing careers in the US.

The Registered Nurse demographics research summary states that currently, as of the printing of the study guide, over 2,904,195 registered nurses (RN) are employed in the US. Most RNs are women (87.7%) and Caucasian (66.1%), followed by African American (11.3%), Asian (9%), Latino (9%), and others (4.6%). The healthcare industry is one area where women and men earn almost at par (94¢ vs. $1). The average wage earned varies from $48,000–$90,000 annually. Most are also in private healthcare industries (Registered Nurse Demographics and Statistics in the US, 2024).

Where would you fall in these statistics regarding nursing? How would you describe your ambitions and goals? Your interest in this guidebook shows that you are an RN or an advanced practice registered nurse (APRN) already working in acute care practices. You want to further your career and earn a specialized certificate to ensure better nursing job prospects or leadership roles.

For many of you, making a critical difference in the lives of others is a reward in itself. Stepping into the acute care hospital setting or as a follow-up for acute care patients, you enter a space where adrenaline flows.

In the US, the American Association of Critical-Care Nurses (AACN) recognizes progressive nursing care as a crucial component of the critical care continuum. It encompasses the collective care of acutely ill patients, spanning emergencies, intermediate care units, direct observation units, stepdown units, telemetry units, and transitional care units. This recognition underscores the significance of your potential role in progressive care.

In all critical care patients, the success of the entire treatment depends on the immediate and aftercare of patients. Even the best medical or surgical procedures fall flat due to a lack of proper post-treatment care. Furthermore, high pressure on the availability of critical care beds and an increasing demand require vacating them sooner than they should be. Patients still require high levels of attention and nursing care; many needing critical care admissions are directly admitted to progressive care units.

To work in a progressive nursing care environment, nurses must have core competency, knowledge, and skills. The Progressive Care Certified Nurse (PCCN) certification ensures that your domain knowledge and skills are up-to-date.

PCCN certifies that you have specialized nursing skills and gives you a sense of pride and accomplishment. PCCN certification will show your dedication to continuous learning and quality care. It may provide a competitive edge for specialty unit positions.

Investing time and effort in your career goals is excellent. But you have a home and career to manage, too. You may have to work overtime and varying shifts.

To pass PCCN, you must study. Working full-time as a nurse makes it challenging to maintain a consistent schedule, especially with overnight shifts or multiple jobs. What resources can help you prepare for the exam? Healthcare-related websites, social media for networking and news, podcasts, and audiobooks can help. But you must know which information you can trust. Which offers exam-oriented information?

Should you solve test questions? Confusion prevails over which will help the most: taking the AACN review course or just answering questions. As you wade through the material, you discover a lot of information that is different from what you deal with regularly. How long should you study, and what can help?

Taking the test and winging it without preparation may not be prudent. These tests provide little scope for guesswork. Repeated failed attempts are disappointing and can lower morale.

This guidebook gives you a complete package where you can revise key theory points. You will also learn the technique to address the final test with our proven *assessment approach,* a unique and structured method to analyze each question on the PCCN exam. This technique has four critical steps:

- Read the question carefully, underlining any key information or clues.
- Identify the primary problem or concern based on the information provided.
- Analyze the answer choices, ruling out any that do not address the primary problem or concern identified in the step.
- Consider each possible action's potential outcomes and identify the best option.

How does this differ from any other exam strategies you have tried before? The systematized and thorough approach mimics the general steps of assessment that you use as a nurse in real-life patient care. Proceeding methodically, you feel more confident about your decision and choice.

The study guide has two sections. Section I is theoretical. It discusses everything you must know for the test.

The Section II is practical. It has three test sets, which are timed and well-designed to resemble the actual test. Section II has question-and-answer components. After finishing your test and scoring it, you can check the answers. Correcting your answers will allow you to reflect, memorize, note, and rework your theory if needed. It should encourage you to explore further reading.

Chapter One: What to Know Before You Start

Data shows that in 2023, out of 3,477 candidates, 70% passed on the first attempt. More than 2,000 new certificates were issued this year (Certification Exam Statistics and Cut Scores, n.d.). What is the secret of those who succeed? The key is to start with a comprehensive idea of the test. It gives you the big-picture approach.

The Cut (Passing) Scores

The cut or the passing score is the number of scored questions you must answer correctly to obtain certification. This number may change depending on the results of the most recent practice study or job analysis. Sometimes, the exam forms are altered and matched for difficulty, causing changes in the passing score.

The passing score must not be confused with the passing percentage or the pass rate. The passing scores for AACN Certification Corporation exams are determined using the systematic Angoff procedure based on professional psychometrics from the PSI testing service. This procedure involves setting a standard for each question and determining how many questions a competent candidate would answer correctly. For example, the PCCN test has 150 questions. There are 125 scored questions. The remaining 25 questions are unscored. For 2024, the passing score is 82, meaning you must correctly answer 82 questions out of 150 (Certification Exam Statistics and Cut Scores, n.d.). It's worth noting that you will not know which questions are scored or unscored.

AACN Certifications

Nurses must be trained to safeguard consumer healthcare. The course programs encompass nursing care and care for acute and critically ill patients. More than 136,000 practicing nurses hold one or more AACN certifications, which can be specialty or subspecialty (Certification Exam Policy Handbook, n.d.). The specialty certificates are:

- The Critical Care Registered Nurse certification (CCRN) ensures that nurses can provide care to or impact the care of acutely or critically ill adult, pediatric, or neonatal patients.
- Progressive Care Certified Nurse certification (PCCN) has two eligibility pathways.

  o Direct care is immediate care to acutely ill adult patients in intermediate care, direct observation, stepdown, telemetry, and transitional care units. You provide direct care to acutely ill adult patients, regardless of location. While renewing your PCCN, opt for the direct care eligibility pathway.
  o Knowledge professionals are the nurses who influence the care delivered to acutely ill adult patients but do not primarily or exclusively provide direct care. Your knowledge will benefit patients, nurses, and organizations in acutely ill patient care. You may have to renew your PCCN via the knowledge professional eligibility pathway.

The Test

Progressive nursing requires caring for moderately stable and acutely ill adult patients with a higher risk of unpredictability. The job analysis, obtained from studying the practice, provides the test basis. It is performed every five years and consists of skills and knowledge necessary for efficient practice as an RN or advanced practice registered nurse (APRN).

An expert PCCN panel makes an exam content outline based on the results of the study of practice. The AACN Synergy Model for Patient Care provides the framework for all AACN certification exams.

Subject matter experts validate clinical practice requirements. The required hours of clinical practice correspond to the third stage of competence in Benner's Stages of Clinical Competence.

Eligibility Criteria

For the direct care pathway, the requirements are:

- A current, unencumbered US RN or APRN license
- Completion of one of the following clinical practice hour requirement options:

  o Two-Year Option: Engaged as an RN or APRN for 1,750 hours in the direct care of acutely/critically ill patients during the previous two years, of which 875 hours must be accumulated in the most recent year before the application.
  o Five-Year Option: You have worked as an RN or APRN during the previous five years, having a minimum of 2,000 hours in the direct care of acutely ill patients. Of these, 144 hours were in the most recent year before the application.

For knowledge professionals, the eligibility criteria for PCCN are:

- A current, unencumbered US RN or APRN license
- Possession of the following practice requirements:

  o Experience as an RN or APRN for 1,040 hours during the previous two years, of which 260 hours are in the most recent year before application. Eligible practice hours are when you use knowledge to help patients, nurses, and organizations care for acutely sick patients and families.
  o Your eligibility criteria concerning clinical practice hours are supported by a professional associate's name and contact information. When selected for audit, this associate must verify in writing that you fulfill the clinical hour requirements. A professional associate is your clinical supervisor, colleague, RN, or physician with whom you work. The

AACN Certification Corporation may have additional eligibility requirements to determine that you have adequate knowledge in caring for the acutely ill for PCCN certification.

PCCN Fees

Exam fees for computer-based tests are $250 for members and $365 for non-members. For retesting, the fees are $175 and $280, respectively. AACN members are engaged in all functions associated with critical care, including intensive care units, progressive care units, cardiac and surgical units, home care, and primary care settings. Their work concerns research, academia, and staff management and development.

Discounts for the test are available for computer-based exams if groups of ten or more candidates submit their AACN certification exam applications in the same envelope. Employers can have further discounted rates for pre-buying exam vouchers.

Application

For computer-based testing, register at www.aacn.org/certification. Processing is completed on the same day. Make sure you have the following documents at hand:

- RN or APRN license number and expiration date
- Name, address, phone, and email address of a professional colleague (RN or physician) or your clinical supervisor who will verify your work eligibility
- Credit card: Visa, MasterCard, Discover, or American Express

A paper application is suitable for candidates appearing as a group, those who opt for paper-and-pencil exams, and off-shore candidates. After filling out and submitting the application, it takes two to four weeks to process.

Successful applicants will receive a confirmation email from AACN and information on scheduling their exam. You must take the test within the eligibility period, currently 180 days.

The confirmation email from AACN bears a link to schedule your exam appointment. Additionally, the AACN customer dashboard has a "Schedule Exam" link. The link lets you choose your preferred computer-based testing option, the PSI Testing Center, or a live remote proctoring from your computer in a silent location. For details, refer to the Certification Exam Policy Handbook online at www.aacn.org/certhandbooks.

The AACN and PSI coordinate to schedule the exam appointments for pen-and-paper tests or tests outside the US.

The computer-based test results will show on the screen, and a detailed score report will be emailed within 24 hours. You will receive the results of paper-and-pencil exams by mail Eight weeks after the exam. Successful candidates obtain individual wall certificates around four weeks after the results. The certification period is counted from the first day of the month when you have passed the exam and ends in three years. You will receive email notifications for renewal four months before the due renewal date. Even if you do not receive a reminder email, you must renew your certification. Information about this is available at www.aacn.org/certification.

The Synergy Model

The Synergy Model underlines an alignment between patient needs and nurse competencies in obtaining optimal outcomes and nurse satisfaction. The model focuses on context and patient-nurse relationships, allowing nurses to step into broader application within nursing practice.

The PCCN test reflects the Synergy Model based on the most recent AACN Certification Corporation nursing practice study. Also relevant to the test are findings on the nursing care of the adult patient population. More information on the AACN Synergy Model is available on their website.

Test Content

The components of the PCCN are described in the following table. This gradation will help you understand the weightage of each element for the test. There are no negative markings; attempt to answer all the questions.

Component categories	Examination percentage
Clinical Judgment	
Cardiovascular (27%) Pulmonary (17%) Endocrine/Hematology/Neurology/Gastrointestinal/Renal (20%) Musculoskeletal/Multisystem/Psychosocial (16%)	80%
Professional Caring and Ethical Practice	
Advocacy/Moral agency/Caring practices/Response to Diversity/Facilitation of learning (11%) Collaboration/Systems thinking/Clinical inquiry (9%)	20%

Answering Questions with the Assessment Approach

The assessment approach to solving the test is integrated with the tenets of the nursing profession. Nursing care comprises the following steps:

- Assessment: Patient data collection is organized yet flexible and dynamic for each patient. This strategy comprises physiological data like age, gender, vitals, or investigative characteristics and psychological, social, spiritual, economic, and lifestyle elements like smoking, alcohol, etc. For instance, to assess pain in hospitalized patients, nurses must consider the patient's physiological and psychological response and the physical causes and symptoms. Pain responses include resentment against oneself or others, fear, withdrawal, or requesting more mediation.

- Diagnosis: Nursing diagnosis depends on the clinical judgment of a patient's response to potential or real health concerns or requirements. For pain diagnosis, one should consider issues caused by pain, such as anxiety and family conflicts. Pain-related immobility can lead to respiratory infection or inadequate nutrition. Your overarching diagnosis forms the crux of a nursing care plan.
- Results/planning: Plans are based on assessment and evaluation. Now, you formulate the answers to the questions you ask while assessing and diagnosing the patient. Glean the facts to form concepts, such as the patient can take a small volume but more frequent meals or move from the bed to a chair at least thrice a day. You support your choice by thorough analysis and logic.
- Implementation: You carry out the actions planned, both short-term and long-term.
- Reappraisal: Since health-related proceedings are dynamic and evolving, all nurses must reassess and modify their action plans accordingly.

Based on this model, we blend the basic nursing framework with the tested SQ3R technique, helping you approach the PCCN test methodically. Use this approach to study your text well and answer the mock tests.

- Information gathering: Concentrate on all the information the question gives you to arrive at your conclusion.

  o   Organize your thought processes before reading the question.
  o   Read the question, making a clear idea about the subject asked.
  o   Focus on the most critical points and understand the purpose of the question.
  o   Consider any graphics like charts, images, or data in the question carefully.
  o   Acknowledge that you understood the question.

- Look for answers to minute details: Reread and ask yourself pertinent questions, answering them in your mind. An active mind searching for solutions to questions can better formulate the correct choice.
- Form your answers: With your questions in mind, read each component to get definitive answers. Identify new questions.

- Zero in on a solution: Once you have chosen your answers based on data and observations, select the best possible fit.
- Revise: Check your answer and move on to the next question.

The approach may seem like an uphill task, but it will become second nature with practice. That is the purpose of this study guide: to develop a habit of reading the text carefully, breaking it into smaller sections, and asking yourself questions as you read. Try to answer these questions from memory based on what you have read. Proceed after you can answer.

Before moving to the next section, recall your questions and answers from memory. It will solidify your concepts.

Follow the same process when answering the questions in the practice tests. Check your answers and read up on the theory to validate them. Consult additional information related to the question. Linking correlated information helps us remember the facts better. Apply the assessment approach tool as we proceed to the theory section on knowledge review.

Section I:
Clinical Judgment

Chapter Two:
Cardiovascular System

PCCN test takers emphasize cardiovascular conditions, assigning them maximum weightage. Cardiovascular diseases (CVD) are the leading cause of death for Americans of most races and ethnicities (Multiple Cause of Death Data, 2023). From 2018 to 2019, heart disease cost the nation about $239.9 billion, including the cost of health services, medicines, and productivity loss due to premature mortality (Heart Disease and Stroke Statistics Update Fact Sheet, 2023).

Aging is an *independent CVD risk factor* compounded by obesity, diabetes, or infirmity. The risk for cardiovascular diseases is lower for women than for age-matched men. Women in their reproductive period have the protective effects of female hormones, estrogen and progesterone. Nevertheless, despite hormone replacement therapy for menopausal and post-menopausal women, the risks and outcomes in women increase with aging (Rodgers, 2019).

The following table shows the American Heart Association (AHA) statistics for the age-specific incidence of CVD in US men and women.

Age group	Incidence of CVD
40–59 years	40%
60–79 years	75%
80 years above	86%

An anticipated two-to-three-fold rise in an aging population by 2050 underscores why understanding heart disease causes, features, and management is vital for adult care nursing.

Hypertension is asignificant CVD risk factor. It is linked to alcohol consumption, poor dietary habits, smoking, and obesity. In older adults, female gender, aging, and obesity are more related to hypertension. An estimated 122.4 million adults ≥ 20 years of age have high blood pressure, more males than females up to 64. The percentage of females with hypertension was higher than for males ≥ 65 years of age.

The Centers for Disease Control and Prevention (CDC) states coronary artery disease (CAD) is the most common type of heart condition (Heart Disease and Stroke Statistics, 2023). Myocardial infarction (MI) is more common in older males than females. However, it could be due to underreporting in females. *One in five heart attacks is silent* (Heart Disease Facts, 2023).

Another major risk for sudden cardiac death that increases with aging is cardiac rhythm abnormalities. Persistent atrial fibrillation (AFib) was found in around 10% of the outpatient population aged 66-93 years old. The incidence of AFib-induced stroke increases from 1.5% in 50–59 years to 23.5% in the 80-89 age group (Wolf et al., 1991).

The average age of patients admitted to the intensive care unit (ICU) is around 60 years; a higher prevalence of elderly ICU patients may show increased rates of heart failure, arrhythmia, and valvular heart disease (Rodgers et al., 2019). We need more specialized units like coronary care units (CCU) or complex procedures and maintenance like mechanical ventilation.

Nursing for these patients requires domain knowledge, skills, and delivering efficient aftercare advice about lifestyle modifications. This chapter discusses symptoms, causes/risk factors, diagnosis, interventions/treatments, complications, and evaluation of different types of CVD.

Acute Coronary Syndrome (ACS)

Myocardial infarction (MI) is a specific diagnosis that doesn't signify one particular cause. When MI is due to acute *atherosclerotic plaque abnormalities* causing *coronary artery thrombosis (atherothrombosis)*, the diagnosis is *ACS*. It can be classified into the following types:

1. Non-segment elevation MI (NSTEMI)
2. ST-segment elevation MI (STEMI)

Both NSTEMI and STEMI are ECG findings of *coronary artery obstruction* due to *atherothrombotic disease*. They are only used to describe *ACS or Type I MI.*

Atherothrombosis

Lipids, fibrous debris, and minerals like calcium obstruct the coronary artery lumen, narrowing vessel walls. Ulceration, fissuring, or erosion can cause thrombus development, which can be silent. Aherothrombosis can cause a heart attack or stroke, increasing morbidity, mortality, and productivity. Paralysis and functional loss may ensue with stroke.

NSTEMI vs. STEMI

NSTEMI is a type of MI due to the complete blockage of a *minor heart artery* or a *major artery* being partially blocked. STEMI, the classic heart attack, is due to the complete occlusion of a major coronary artery by atherothrombosis, causing extensive myocardial damage.

In the US, the median age of NSTEMI is 68 years, with male dominance. Most patients presenting with ACS in the US show NSTEMI (Goyal & Zeltser, 2022). NSTEMI causes myocardial damage and is considered a heart attack (MI) with a better prognosis than STEMI. Unlike STEMI, NSTEMI affects not the major coronary but the tiny collaterals, causing *diffuse coronary disease*.

Unstable Angina

Unstable angina is similar to NSTEMI and causes chest discomfort and pain due to insufficient blood and oxygen flow to the heart.

Acute MI

MI damages the myocardium (heart muscle), which raises cardiac troponin values above the 99th percentile upper reference limit with a changeable rise/fall over time. With this, there must be at least two clinical evidence of MI, such as:

1. Anginal symptoms
2. An electrocardiogram (ECG) shows new ischemic changes or left bundle branch block (LBBB)
3. Pathological Q waves on ECG
4. Echocardiography shows new regional wall motion abnormality or ischemic loss of healthy myocardium
5. Angiographic or autopsy evidence of coronary thrombus

MI causes *irreversible damage to the cardiac muscle* due to lack of oxygen. It impairs systolic and diastolic heart functions, increasing the risks of arrhythmias and other complications.

The aim is to establish blood flow and reperfusion of heart tissues. Treatments started early, *before six hours of symptom onset*, have a better prognosis.

Pathophysiology

Rupture of atherosclerotic plaques causes 70% of cases of MI (ACS or Type I MI) due to plaque thrombosis and acute occlusion of blood vessels. Decreased coronary blood flow leads to low oxygen perfusion to the myocardium, causing cardiac ischemia. Other causes of MI are coronary artery embolism, cocaine, coronary dissections, and coronary vasospasm.

Risk

Modifiable risk factors account for 90% of MI in men and 94% in women and include cigarette smoking, exercise, hypertension, obesity, cholesterol, LDL, and triglyceride levels. Age, gender, and family history are non-modifiable risk factors for atherosclerosis.

Symptoms

History-taking includes onset, duration, nature, pain radiation, and associated features. Sweating and pain radiation are more common in males. Other symptoms also include:

1. Dizziness
2. Anxiousness
3. Choking sensations
4. Profuse sweating
5. Respiratory difficulties
6. Irregular heart rates

Signs

Taking patients' vitals, noting their appearance (anxiousness, pallor, etc.), lung and heart findings are parts of physical exams. Note the following:

1. High blood pressure (BP). Low in shock.
2. Unequal pulses in aortic dissection.
3. Heart rate may show tachycardia (> 100 beats/minutes at rest), atrial fibrillation, or ventricular arrhythmia.
4. Distended neck veins showing right heart failure.
5. Tachypnea (rapid shallow breathing) and fever.
6. Cardiac palpation reveals lateral displacement of apical impulse, soft S1, palpable S4, and new mitral regurgitation murmur. Ventricular rupture can be indicated by a loud holosystolic murmur radiating to the sternum.
7. Chest auscultation shows wheezing and rales (clicking or rattling lung sounds on inhalation), indicating pulmonary edema.

8. Extremities can be cold and blue (cyanosis) due to inadequate tissue perfusion.

Diagnosis

1. Presence of consistent symptoms and physical findings: Women and diabetic patients may have atypical symptoms like abdominal pain or vomiting without definitive chest pain.
2. ECG is 97% specific for MI, with 30% sensitivity. Sensitivity increases with right-sided, posterior lead placement and repeat testing. ST-elevations > 2 mm in two adjacent leads on ECG (inferior: leads II, III, aVF; septal: V1, V2; anterior: V3, V4; lateral: I, aVL, V5, V6) indicate STEMI.

    a. ECG diagnosis of STEMI in patients with LBBB or pacemakers is difficult. In these settings, isolated ST-elevation in aVR means left main coronary artery occlusion in appropriate clinical features (Sgarbosa technique). Biphasic T waves in V2 and V3 often predict an impending proximal left anterior descending artery occlusion. It can lead to massive anterior wall myocardial infarction (Wellens technique).

    b. NSTEMI ECG may lack acute changes or have subtle changes. Serial ECG can be helpful.

3. Elevated cardiac troponin.
4. Clinician's *hunch*, *ECG* findings, patient's *age* and *risk factors*, and *troponin* levels (HEART score) determine their risks for short-term adverse outcomes from ACS.

Management

Immediately stabilize the patient with oxygen, morphine, nitrates, beta blockers, aspirin, and statins. STEMI needs immediate perfusion by percutaneous coronary intervention (PCI). PCI within 48 hours of admission may have improved outcomes and reduced length of stay. The patient is primed with dual antiplatelet agents—intravenous (IV) heparin infusion and an adenosine diphosphate receptor (P2Y2) inhibitor. All patients receive parenteral anticoagulation and antiplatelet therapy. Patients are discharged on aspirin, high-dose statin, beta-blocker, and/or ACE inhibitors.

If PCI is unavailable within 90 minutes of STEMI diagnosis, reperfusion with an intravenous thrombolytic agent is attempted. Stable and asymptomatic NSTEMI receive antiplatelet agents only.

Nursing Care Plan

A thorough assessment creates *an accurate nursing diagnosis* and *an appropriate care plan* (Martin, 2023).

Assessment

1. Daily ECG
2. Cardiac enzyme monitoring
3. Vitals and pulse oximetry
4. Patients with cardiac catheters are checked for hematoma in the groin and distal femoral pulses.

Diagnosis

Nursing diagnosis differs from medical diagnosis in *analyzing patients' responses to their health conditions or diseases.* It focuses on changes associated with dynamic patient needs. In MI, relevant nursing diagnoses are:

1. Acute pain
2. Intolerance to activity
3. Anxiety or fear
4. Risks for diminished cardiac output
5. Risks for inadequate tissue perfusion
6. Risks for fluid overload
7. Inadequate knowledge

Interventions

1. The patient must always have two large-bore intravenous (IV) channels
2. Initiation of treatment for acute MI
3. Morphine administration for pain
4. Immediate aspirin and 0.4 mg sublingual nitroglycerin
5. Oxygen if pulse oximetry is < 94% at room air
6. Cardiologist referral and ensuring it is done
7. Regular checks of vitals, urine output, and daily weight checks
8. Heparin, as per order for STEMI

Seek Help

1. Hypotension (BP fall)
2. Nausea/vomiting
3. Persistent chest pain
4. Unable to find distal leg pulses (emboli or low blood pressure)
5. A sudden change in mental awareness
6. Oxygen desaturation persisting
7. Tachycardia/arrhythmias
8. Sudden loud murmur (new-onset mitral regurgitation or ventricular rupture)

Desired Outcome

1. Breathing improvement
2. Chest pain alleviation
3. Tissue perfusion improvement
4. Functional restoration as before

Evaluation

1. ECG
2. Cardiac enzymes
3. Oxygenation-pulse oximetry

4. Vital signs
5. Chest pain intensity
6. Leg pulses
7. Chest auscultation for rales and new murmurs

Care Coordination

A solely dedicated cardiac interprofessional team manages MI. It comprises a cardiologist, interventional cardiologist, cardiac surgeon, intensivist, critical care or cardiology nurses, cardiac rehabilitation specialist, and physical therapists.

High morbidity and mortality rates require health providers to educate patients about MI symptoms and early hospital care. The pharmacist, nurse practitioner, and primary care physicians advise patients to *call 911 after three nitroglycerin doses if they don't feel better.*

The nurse must promptly notify the interprofessional team at triage for quick reperfusion. Nurses must note and inform for life-threatening complications.

MI complications can arise a week after the occurrence, precluding premature discharge. The nurse thoroughly informs stable patients about minimizing coronary heart disease risk and plans cardiac rehab and home care with a social worker. Pharmacists answer drug questions and examine side effects.

Evidence-based findings are:

1. A prognosis is best with early intervention.
2. Fewer risk factors improve outcomes.

Prognosis

About a third of the patients die before arrival at the hospital. Upon arrival, mortality is as high as 40%–50%; 5%–10% of patients will die within the first 12 months after MI. Readmission occurs in about 50% of patients within 12 months after the initial MI (Mechanic et al., 2023). The prognosis depends on the ejection fraction, age, and other associated comorbidity. Prognosis is best in patients with early and successful reperfusion and preserved left ventricular function; prognosis is poorer without revascularization procedures.

Acute Cardiac Inflammatory Disease

Myocarditis

Myocarditis is a self-limiting, acute inflammation of the myocardium. It can cause arrhythmias, pericarditis, chronic dilated cardiomyopathy, and heart failure (HF).

Causes

1. Infective

    a. Viral infections trigger an autoimmune response, prolonging inflammation and damaging heart muscle.

        i. Coxsackievirus and echovirus are the most common
        ii. Human immunodeficiency virus (HIV)
        iii. Rubella or rubeola (in children)
        iv. Herpes simplex
        v. Influenza
        vi. Hepatitis B or C
        vii. Cytomegalovirus (CMV)
        viii. Epstein-Barr virus (EB-virus)

    b. Bacterial

        i. Staphylococci
        ii. Salmonella
        iii. Shigella
        iv. Streptococci
        v. Clostridium
        vi. Tuberculosis

     c. Parasites

        i.   Trichinosis
       ii.   Schistosomiasis

     d. Protozoa

        i.   Trypanosoma cruzi (Chagas disease)
       ii.   Toxoplasmosis gondii

     e. Spirochetes

        i.   Borrelia burgdorferi

2. Non-infective

     a. Autoimmune diseases such as lupus, ulcerative colitis, and rheumatoid arthritis
     b. Allergic response to medications, chemotherapy, and radiation therapy
     c. Chemical exposures

3. Pregnancy and aging
4. Idiopathic (No known causes)

Symptoms

1. Mild cases show vague symptoms of viral infections, such as headache, myalgia, and fatigue.
2. Sharp stabbing precordial pain/ substernal squeezing pain similar to MI.
3. Dyspnea (shortness of breath) on exertion and palpitations
4. Dyspnea at rest, cough, and feet edema in patients with heart failure.

Diagnosis

Usually, the initial viral infection abates when patients present with myocarditis.

Patient history and physical examination help with diagnosis. Differentiation from MI in cases of chest pain is crucial.

1. ECG
2. An echocardiogram (cardiac ultrasound) showing:

    a. Left ventricular dysfunction and its degree
    b. Congenital defects
    c. Pericardial effusion
    d. Cardiac tamponade

3. Blood cultures and an increased white blood cell count may suggest a recent infection. Serum viral titers can identify the pathogen.
4. Serum cardiac biomarkers (troponin I) to identify myocardial damage.

5. Cardiac catheterization with endo-myocardial biopsy can be a definitive diagnosis.

Nursing Care Plan

1. Bed rest reduces the heart's workload. Monitor the patient carefully for arrhythmias and treat them according to the order. Regular physical assessments help identify signs and symptoms of heart failure.
2. Depending on the severity of the condition and damage to the myocardium, the patient may fully recover or develop chronic heart failure. During discharge, explain any diet or exercise restrictions and educate the patient on recognizing the signs and symptoms of heart failure. Inform them to contact their cardiologist or dial 911 immediately for worsening symptoms.

Endocarditis

Endocarditis is inflammation of the inner lining of the heart's chambers and valves or endocardium. The condition has high mortality if left untreated.

Pathophysiology

The endocardium becomes infected when pathogens enter the bloodstream (bacteremia) from elsewhere. It can happen after operations, dental procedures, or serious illnesses when a sudden bacteria load enters the bloodstream. Biological colonies can grow on valves damaged by rheumatic fever, congenital valve defects, or on mechanical heart valves. Microorganism colonization provokes inflammation, forming "vegetations" of bacteria, platelets, fibrin, and inflammatory cells on the valves.

Vegetation destroys heart valves, causing regurgitation or stenosis. In regurgitation, valves fail to close during ventricular contraction, and blood flow leaks, while in stenosis, narrowing valves prevent blood from entering the arteries. Impaired perfusion hampers tissue oxygenation. Heart failure can result from overloading.

Vegetations may break off into emboli (embolus). They travel through the bloodstream, blocking smaller blood vessels and causing stroke and organ dysfunction. Infected emboli can lodge in distant foci, such as the lungs or spleen, causing classic but non-specific infective symptoms such as fever, fatigue, and raised heart rate or organ-specific symptoms such as dyspnea, chest pain, and cough.

Causes

1. Infections

    a. Bacterial infections—Streptococcus and Staphylococcus species—are the main cause of infective endocarditis. Individuals with pre-existing heart conditions are more susceptible.
    b. Fungal infections, particularly Candida species, in individuals with weak immune systems.

2. Intravenous drug use with non-sterile needles can inject bacteria directly into the bloodstream. Endocarditis occurrence has risen among people with opioid use disorder. A spike between 2021 and 2022 could be due to the Covid-19 pandemic (Facher, 2023).

3. Structural heart abnormalities.
4. Procedures and surgeries, such as dental work or surgeries of the respiratory or gastrointestinal tracts in predisposing patients.

Symptoms

1. Chest pain
2. Heart failure symptoms

Signs

1. Raised temperature
2. Raised white blood cell (WBC)
3. HF signs
4. Murmurs
5. Diminished Saturation of peripheral oxygen (SpO2)
6. Embolic complications

   a. Splinter hemorrhages in nail beds
   b. Janeway lesions on fingers, toes, nose
   c. Clubbing of fingers

Nursing Care Plan

Assessment

1. Clinical history: medical history of recent infections, dental procedures, or intravenous drug use
2. Symptom: fever, fatigue, new or changed heart murmurs, and signs of emboli
3. Cardiovascular: auscultation for murmurs, heart sounds, and signs of heart failure or embolic events.
4. Systemic signs: clubbing, Janeway lesions, Osler nodes, or Roth spots
5. Laboratory tests: blood cultures, complete blood count (CBC), inflammatory markers [erythrocyte sedimentation rate (ESR) and C-reactive protein(CRP)], and cardiac biomarkers

6. Echocardiography: heart valve, vegetation, and the extent of involvement visualization
7. Renal function: serum creatinine and blood urea nitrogen (BUN)
8. Neurological: focal neurological deficits/changes in mental status (emboli), headaches, seizures, or toxic encephalopathy

Interventions

1. Prompt, appropriate, and prolonged IV antibiotic therapy based on blood culture reports and susceptibility
2. IV fluids for adequate hydration, cardiac output, and perfusion
3. Fluid rate monitoring, especially with heart failure risks
4. Pain management with prescribed analgesics without compromising cardiovascular stability
5. Continuous monitoring and support of vital signs, cardiac function, and oxygen saturation
6. Respiratory support, including supplemental oxygen or mechanical ventilation
7. Cardiac team guidance when necessary
8. Surgical intervention like valve repair or replacement for severe valvular damage or persistent infection despite antibiotic therapy

The following table shows nursing interventions and rationalities.

Interventions

Interventions	Rationale
Assess heart sounds.	Heart murmurs or extra sounds.
Address oral hygiene.	Oral bacteria can reach the heart. To avoid problems, all hospitalized patients (even surgical patients) should brush twice a day.
Administer IV antibiotics.	Specific antibiotics treat bacterial infections. IV works faster.
Administer and monitor anticoagulant therapy.	Prevent the collection of platelets or clots around the valves and check emboli formation. IV heparin needs partial thromboplastin time (PTT) monitoring.

Interventions	Rationale
Apply thromboembolic deterrent stockings (TEDS) and sequential compression devices (SCDs) to prevent deep vein thrombosis (DVT).	DVT is the most common cause of pulmonary embolism.
Assess for systemic emboli; the common sites are pulmonary, retina, and brain.	Emboli can cause stroke, MI, and pulmonary, retinal, and limb embolisms.

Desired Outcome

1. Endocarditis-causing bacteria elimination, inflammatory markers and cardiac biomarkers normalization are *infection and inflammation control.*
2. Valvular function restoration prevents insufficiency and stenosis.
3. Infection control reduces the risk of emboli, septicemia, and organ damage.
4. Relief of fever, tiredness, and heart symptoms.

Patient Education

Infection prevention is curative.

1. Inform the patient about infection prevention, such as hand cleanliness and notifying infections, such as skin, teeth, nails, etc.
2. Alert the patient to tell other doctors about prophylactic antibiotics before surgery.
3. Endocarditis patients should wait 6 months for dental work.

Pericarditis

Pericarditis is inflammation of the outer double-layered sac of the heart and the roots of major blood vessels. It is accompanied by an increase in normally serous (serum-like) and scant pericardial fluid.

Depending on onset and progress, pericarditis can be acute, subacute, or chronic. Acute pericarditis happens suddenly and resolves completely within three weeks. It may recur.

Subacute pericarditis with persistent symptoms lasts six weeks, not exceeding three months. Chronic pericarditis with a slow onset lasts more than three months.

Causes

The majority of cases are idiopathic (90%). Heart attack or surgery can cause pericarditis, known as Dressler syndrome. Other causes can be infective or non-infective.

1. Infective: infection anywhere in the body can trigger an inflammatory response in the pericardium, especially in compromised hosts.

   a. Viruses: coxsackieviruses A and B, echovirus, adenoviruses, parvovirus B19, HIV, influenza
   b. Bacteria: tuberculosis
   c. Fungus in immunocompromised individuals

2. Non-infective

   a. Malignancy
   b. Connective tissue disease
   c. Trauma: heart surgery
   d. Medications

Symptoms

The symptoms of pericarditis depend on the volume and speed of pericardial fluid accumulation (*pericardial effusion*). In a slowly progressing disease, symptoms may not show despite a large volume of pericardial fluid.

1. Chest pain is a *common symptom* associated with pericarditis.

   a. Sharp and stabbing pain/dull and pressure-like
   b. Under the breastbone/the left side of the chest

    c. Radiation along the left arm

    d. Relieved by sitting up and leaning forward

4. Abdominal/leg swelling
5. Cough
6. Generalized weakness
7. Palpitations
8. Mild fever
9. Dyspnea on lying down

Complications

1. *Cardiac tamponade* is a life-threatening complication needing immediate medical attention. A massive quantity of fluid puts pressure on the heart, preventing its pumping function and causing blood pressure to fall.
2. *Chronic constrictive pericarditis* is permanent scarring of the pericardium that affects heart pumping.

Diagnosis

1. History of fever, chest pain, trauma, heart attack, etc. Determine acute, subacute, or chronic.
2. Physical examination, including muffled heart sound auscultation. The sound of pericardial layers rubbing is called a friction rub.
3. Blood and urine testing can diagnose cause of pericarditis.
4. An ECG.
5. Chest X-rays assess heart size, shape, and effusion.
6. An echocardiography measures pumping ability.
7. Chest computed tomography (CT) scans reveal the heart's shape and size, suggest restrictive pericarditis, and rule out other heart disorders.
8. Magnetic resonance imaging (MRI) scan of the chest is helpful when the other forms of imaging are inconclusive.

Management

The cause determines treatment; some diseases resolve on their own.

1. Pericarditis medication can alleviate symptoms.
2. Medications to relieve pain.
3. Anti-gout medications.
4. Corticosteroids minimize inflammation.
5. Pericardiocentesis involves ultrasound-guided aspiration of pericardial fluid. The fluid is tested in tumor, malignancy, and trauma labs.
6. Constrictive pericarditis requires pericardiectomy (removal of the pericardium).

Nursing Care Plan

Diminished Cardiac Output (CO)

Assessment

Fatigue and incapacity to perform ADLs indicate decreased CO (Curran, 2022).

The following table explains nursing interventions and rationalities.

Interventions	Rationale
Check the patient's heartbeat and vitals every four hours. Listen to heartbeats. Slow capillary refill, face pallor, cyanosis, and chilly, clammy skin indicate reduced peripheral tissue perfusion and diminished CO.	A new or changing heart murmur suggests pericarditis. Reduced peripheral tissue perfusion suggests deterioration and demands urgent medical treatment.
Administer prescribed antibiotics.	Antibiotics treat bacterial infections.
Administer supplemental oxygen as ordered. Discontinue if the SpO2 level exceeds the target range or per physician's orders.	To raise the oxygen level and achieve targeted SpO2 value.

Interventions	Rationale
Instruct the patient on stress management, deep breathing, and relaxation.	Chronic stress produces cortisol, and adrenaline, raising HR, respiration, and blood sugar. Managing fatigue requires stress reduction.
Make the patient ready for surgical interventions.	Removing fluid by needle aspiration from the pericardial sac is called pericardiocentesis. Pericardiectomy removes the pericardium for constrictive pericarditis.

Desirable Outcome

The patient will have enough CO to participate in ADLs and feel better.

Acute Chest Pain

Interventions

The following table explains nursing interventions and rationalities.

Intervention	Rationale
Check the patient's vitals. Ask the patient to rate and describe their pain on a scale of 0 to 10.	Establish baseline observations. Worldwide, the 10-point pain scale is precise and effective.
Administer recommended painkillers. Give antibiotics as directed.	Treats discomfort and infection.
Ask the patient to rate acute pain 30–60 minutes after analgesics.	Medication effectiveness review.
Interventions	Rationale
At prescribed intervals, provide more analgesics as needed.	Pain and discomfort alleviation without overdosing.
Raise the bedhead and encourage the patient to sit semi-Fowler. Promote pursed lips and deep breathing.	To reduce breathlessness and expand lungs, maximize patient comfort, and alleviate anxiety/restlessness.

Desirable Outcome

A patient will have a pain score of 0 out of 10.

Aneurysm

An aortic aneurysm is an abnormal dilation of the aortic wall due to localized weakness and stretching of the medial muscular layer of the artery. The aorta is a major artery arising out of the left side of the ventricle of the heart. An aortic aneurysm can be as follows:

1. Abdominal aortic aneurysm (AAA): along the descending branch of the aorta.
2. Thoracic aortic aneurysm (TAA): in the ascending part of the aorta. Individuals with Marfan syndrome can have a TAA.

Treatment aims at modifying the risk factors to limit disease progression. The prognosis is poor for a ruptured aneurysm, requiring immediate surgery.

1. BP control (relieves aneurysm pressure).
2. Early symptom detection.
3. Rupture prevention.

Investigations

1. Chest X-ray, angiogram, MRI, and transesophageal echocardiography (TEE).
2. Duplex ultrasonography/CT.

   While waiting on the surgery, medical measures include:

Surgery

Surgery removes the aneurysm and restores vascular flow with a graft. Resection and bypass graft or endovascular grafting are the treatments of choice (TOC) for AAA larger than two inches in diameter or increasing aneurysms. CCU care requires intensive monitoring in the postoperative period.

Pharmacologic Highlights

1. Opioid analgesic (morphine) 1–10 mg IV to relieve surgical pain.
2. Opioid analgesic (Fentanyl) 50–100 mcg IV to relieve surgical pain.
3. Antihypertensives/diuretics for elevated BP to reduce stress on graft suture lines.
4. Beta-blocker (propranolol) 80–400 mg/day in divided doses to reduce cardiac contractility and pulsatile flow to the aneurysm.

Nursing Care Plan

Assessment

1. Prominent, pulsating mass in the abdomen, at or above the umbilicus
2. Systolic bruit over the aorta
3. Tenderness on deep palpation
4. Abdominal/lower back pain

Diagnosis

1. Fluid volume deficit due to hemorrhage is the prime risk.
2. Other diagnoses include the following:

   a. Decreased CO related to

      i. Alteration in intravascular volume
      ii. Raised systemic vascular resistance
      iii. Elevated third-space fluid shift (hemorrhagic shock)

   b. Acute pain due to surgical tissue trauma
   c. Anxiety regarding a threat to health. The type of aneurysm determines the nature of the treatment, whether medical or surgical.

Interventions

1. Adjust risk factors.
2. Inform the patient about the need for frequesnt BP monitoring. Systolic blood pressure (SBP) must be maintained at 100–120 mm Hg.
3. Encourage the patient to see the doctor routinely to monitor the aneurysm.
4. Inform the patient to promptly report significant back or stomach pain or fullness, umbilicus tenderness, sudden extremities discoloration, or persistently elevated BP to the doctor.
5. Tell a patient with TAA to report chest/back pain, shortness of breath, swallowing difficulties, or hoarseness.

Evaluation

1. Vital signs.
2. Risk factors for progression of the arterial disease process.
3. Back or abdominal pain.
4. Abdominal sensation on palpation.
5. Skin for the presence of vascular disease or breakdown.
6. Peripheral circulation, including pulses, temperature, and color.
7. Signs of rupture.
8. Tenderness over the abdomen.
9. Abdominal distention.

Documentation

1. What soothes pain, its location, intensity, and frequency?
2. Note the abdominal wound's appearance, color, warmth, integrity, and drainage.
3. Verify vital signs, hydration, bowel sounds, and electrolyte stability.
4. Complications include hypotension, hypertension, cardiac dysrhythmias, reduced urine output, thrombophlebitis, infection, graft blockage, consciousness changes, aneurysm rupture, extreme anxiety, or poor wound healing.

Patient Education on Discharge

1. Surgical wound care

    a. Keep it dry and clean.
    b. Report redness, swelling, drainage, odor, or wound edge separation.
    c. Report a fever.

2. Activity limit

    a. Lift no more than 5 pounds for 6–12 weeks.
    b. Avoid driving until the doctor approves. Braking while driving can damage the suture line and raise intra-abdominal pressure.
    c. Advise against pushes, pulls, or stretches (vacuuming, changing linens, playing tennis and golf, trimming grass, and cutting wood).

3. Encourage the patient to quit smoking and attend addiction treatment.
4. Inform about clots and graft blockage.
5. Ensure treatment and follow-up compliance. Emphasize understanding of antihypertensive medications.
6. Instruct to report abdominal fullness or back pain, which may suggest a rupture.

Cardiac Surgery

Coronary artery bypass graft (CABG), cardiac valve surgeries, and aortic procedures are the most common cardiac operations in the US.

Cardiopulmonary bypass (CPB) in the 1950s shaped modern cardiac surgical procedures. The use of "off-pump" approaches, especially for CABG, is rising. Post-CABG ICU issues cause the most fatalities.

Types of Cardiac Surgery

Closed Heart Surgery

Mitral valvotomy is the most common closed heart surgery done through a thoracotomy. Access to the heart is through a cut on the ventricular/atrial wall. The stenosed valve is dilated with a special balloon catheter. The balloon valvuloplasty technique avoids thoracotomy and is performed in the cardiac cath lab. The costly procedure cuts hospital stays. Other examples of closed heart surgery are pericardiectomy and repairing minor heart defects.

Open Heart Surgery

Surgeons access the heart through the sternum and spread the ribs, requiring CPB to continue systemic perfusion of oxygenated blood during heart operation. Common open heart procedures are:

1. *Open mitral valvotomy* in mitral stenosis.
2. *Annuloplasty* in mitral regurgitation and tricuspid regurgitation.
3. *Valve replacement* surgeries (changing the diseased valve with biological tissue valves or mechanical valves).
4. *Coronary artery bypass graft* in coronary artery block.
5. *Thoracic aortic aneurysm resection.*
6. *Excision* of fibrous tissue or myxoma.

Other Cardiac Surgeries

1. *Heart transplant*: a healthy donor's heart replaces the damaged one.
2. *Pacemaker or ICD implantation:* for arrhythmia if medical management fails. Sensors detect abnormal heart rhythms that the pacemaker manages.
3. *Maze surgery* for atrial fibrillation is the most frequent severe arrhythmia. Scar tissue is built in the upper heart chambers to divert electrical signals to the lower heart chambers.

ICU Care

The cardiac surgical ICU is usually connected to the operation theater. It facilitates patient transport in and out of the surgery for postoperative complications (bleeding or cardiac tamponade).

Preparation of the Unit

The ICU, including the ICU bed and other equipment, is cleaned and sanitized thoroughly.

All equipment must be ready at hand or readily accessible. These include a cardiac monitor with all the cables, a ventilator with sterile water in a humidifier, central suction for endotracheal suction and low suction system to connect the chest drainage system, an arterial flush system with the transducers set in order, drainage bottle bags for gastric drainage, central oxygen supply for ventilator, IV pole hangers, syringes, needles, emergency drugs, emergency cart with sterile pack sets to meet any emergency, defibrillator, and pacemakers.

Prepare the flow charts; ICU special charts are unique for each hospital's cardiac unit. The chart maintains the complete records of activities and events in the ICU. It includes hourly inputs of administered fluids such as blood, plasma, other colloids and crystalloids, hourly chest drainage in each drainage bottle, hourly gastric drainage, hourly urine output, hourly monitoring of arterial blood gas analysis, serum electrolyte, glucose, and vitals like pulse, heart rate, respiratory rate, and mean BP. The chart also mentions medications given and the nurses' notes.

A mean arterial pressure (MAP) of 60–90 mm Hg and a systolic blood pressure of 90–140 mm Hg are considered safe. Warm extremities with strong pulses and good urine output (≥ 0.5 ml/kg/hr) assure adequate perfusion supported by objective data. Crystalloids are preferred for fluid resuscitation.

Immediate Post-Op Care

The immediate postoperative period, from 2 to 72 hours, is critical. A surgeon, anesthetist, and the nurse who assists with the surgery accompany the patient to the ICU with a portable ventilator and ECG monitor. Perform the following:

1. Transfer the patient to the bed.
2. Attach the ECG leads to the cardiac monitor.
3. Fix the pressure lines, the central venous pressure (CVP), left atrial pressure (LAP), and arterial BP lines to the flush system. Hourly readings and monitoring are a must.
4. Connect the ventilator to the endotracheal (ET) tube after ET suction. Set the parameters and assess their functions.
5. Determine respiratory rate and record. Assess breath sounds to ensure the endotracheal tube is placed correctly and both lungs are aerated. Repeat ET suction hourly, perform chest physiotherapy, and change the patient's position to promote ventilation and perfusion of the lungs.
6. The chest drainages are hooked to the central suction. Milk the tubes to assess chest tube patency. Suspect hemorrhage if the drainage is above 70 ml/hr from individual tubes and the color is red and free-flowing. Continue milking the chest tubes hourly. Monitor the amount and color and record them on the flow chart.
7. Fix the urinary bag to the bed, measure the urine in the bag. Diuretics may be prescribed if urine output is less than 0.5 ml/kg/hr (oliguria).
8. Release the gastric drainage tube and record the amount and color of drainage.
9. Connect the temperature probe and pulse oximetry to the monitor.
10. Check and adjust IV lines, fluid volumes in the bottles, and drip rates.
11. Monitor hourly blood gasses for the first 12 hours, then every two hours.
12. Arrange for chest X-rays as advised.
13. Reassure the patient that the operation is over and that they are in ICU. Make them feel comfortable.
14. The patient is weaned off the ventilator gradually if no complications occur, breathing is effective, and arterial blood gas (ABG) is normal.
15. Give proper mouthwash after extubation.
16. Continue humidified oxygen inhalation using a venturi mask, monitor ABG every four hours, cup, clap, vibrate, and turn position hourly depending on the cardiac status.

17. Weaning off the patient from respiratory support is usually possible within 48–72 hours. Continue two hourly breathing exercises when the patient is awake. Keep support on the sternal incision area with a folded soft towel or small pillow.

18. Steam inhalation helps bring out the secretion.

19. Assess chest dressing for any soakage and bulging. Document and report immediately.

20. Remove the chest drainage when the drainage volume is less than 50 ml/24 hours.

21. Encourage ambulation. Serous drainage may continue sometimes. The patient can ambulate with the chest drainage tubes, which are removed once drainage reduces.

22. Observe any life-threatening dysrhythmia. Repeat serum sodium and potassium two hours daily for 12 hours and then four to six hours daily. Reduced (hypokalemia) and raised (hyperkalemia) potassium can cause dysrhythmia. Keep a defibrillator ready to use at the bedside.

23. Administer the prescribed inotropes dopamine or dobutamine IV infusion in the immediate post-op period. In the 24–72 hours post-op, arterial lines are flushed at regular intervals with heparin. Monitor 12 lead ECG daily. With stabilization, the patient is weaned off the pressure lines and vasodilator or vasopressor drugs. The arterial pressure line, LA catheter, and CVP are removed. The pressure dressing is applied to the arterial puncture site. Pacing wires remain in place. Hemoglobin (Hb) and hematocrit values are checked daily.

24. Start a small oral feed after weaning off the ventilator. If the patient tolerates it, give light fluids in a small amount, and then a light semi-solid meal. Document the intake and output in the flow chart in the ICU.

25. Record weight. With stabilization, remove the urinary catheter and other drainage tubes. Infection prevention is paramount in the ICU. All invasive lines have sterile drapes. Broad-spectrum antibiotics are administered through the IV line.

26. Assist the patient with oral hygiene, sponging, and changing clothing.

27. Keep the environment clean, quiet, and calm. Pain-relieving drugs such as IV morphine are given initially. Later, the patient receives oral analgesic drugs to relieve pain in the sternum and other body parts.

28. Monitor psycho-emotional aspects is important. ICU structures aim to reduce sensory deprivation. Communicate with the patient, listen to

them, and encourage them to convey verbally and nonverbally (Nursing Management of Patients with Cardiac Surgery, n.d.).

Cardiac Tamponade

Excess fluid in the pericardial space causes cardiac tamponade, which impairs heart filling and stroke volume and causes coronary artery compression and myocardial ischemia. The clinical signs of cardiac tamponade depend on the speed and amount of fluid accumulation.

Risk Factors

1. Recent cardiac trauma, such as gunshot wounds and stabs, closed trauma (impact of the chest on a steering wheel during a motor vehicle accident)
2. Cardiac surgery
3. Iatrogenic (medical) events like cardiac catheterization or pacemaker electrode perforation

Symptoms

1. Agitation
2. Faintness
3. Chest discomfort
4. Breathing difficulty
5. A feeling of impending death

Signs

1. Pulsus paradoxus > 10 mm Hg (hallmark)
2. Narrowed pulse pressure (< 30 mm Hg)
3. Hypotension
4. Confused and numbed mental state
5. Jugular vein distention in the neck

6. Reflex tachycardia
7. Muffled heart sounds
8. Cool, pale, and clammy extremities

Nursing Care Plan

Priority

Nursing priority determines the crucial aspects of the care plan. In cardiac tamponade, increased pericardial pressure reduces ventricular filling and CO. It is a priority concern. Optimizing CO is essential to improving client outcomes and quality of life.

Assessment

1. Echocardiogram and ECG monitoring for dysrhythmia may indicate myocardial ischemia from epicardial coronary artery compression.
2. Check BP every 5–15 minutes throughout the acute phase.
3. Watch for pulsus paradoxus during arterial tracing or manual BP monitoring.
4. Monitor urine output hourly; a reduction may suggest decreased renal perfusion due to stroke volume reduction.

Interventions

1. Supplemental oxygen.
2. Two large-bore IV lines for fluid administration.
3. Medications like dobutamine to boost myocardial contractility and reduce peripheral vascular resistance.
4. Monitoring and management of dysrhythmias and coronary artery laceration.
5. Surgical interventions to locate and repair the bleeding site, remove mediastinal clots, and resection of the pericardium.

Desired Outcome

1. The patient must be alert and focused.
2. The skin should be warm and dry.
3. Pulses are strong and equal.
4. Capillary refill time is < 3 sec.
5. Heart rate (HR) is 60-100 beats/min.
6. BP is 90–120 mm Hg.
7. Pulse pressure is 30–40 mm Hg.
8. Urine output is 30 ml/hr or 1 ml/kg/hr.

Cardiac/Vascular Catheterization

An invasive cardiac/vascular catheterization operation using a contrast involves inserting a flexible catheter into the heart or blood vessel, usually through the femoral vein. It measures blood gasses, pressures, cardiac output, and anatomical flaws such as septal defects and blockages. Therapeutic cardiac catheterizations use balloon angioplasty to fix stenotic valves, arteries, aortic blockage, and patent ductus arteriosus closure.

Nursing Care Plan

Priorities

1. *Improving tissue perfusion* is vital. Monitoring patients for bleeding, vascular damage, and tissue perfusion helps avert issues.
2. Cardiac catheterization involves aseptic procedures, infection surveillance, and wound care.
3. The procedure's invasiveness, difficulties, and unknown outcomes necessitate fear and anxiety reduction.
4. The following table shows assessments, intervention, and rationalities.

Assessment	Intervention	Rationale
Body temperature regulation	Monitor body temperature six times hourly and use warming blankets or cooling techniques to check hypo or hyperthermia. Record hourly fluid intake and outflow.	Regulating body temperature helps with hemodynamic stability and recovery time. Prevent dehydration or overhydration.
Reduce anxiety	Assess catheterization knowledge and concerns. Explain catheterization processes.	Emotions might impair hemodynamic stability and recovery.
Ensure tissue perfusion	Check the extremity's color, temperature, and capillary refill. Feel distal pulses.	A puncture site clot could block distal blood flow and cause tissue damage.
Sufficient tissue perfusion	Doppler every 15 minutes 4 times, 30 minutes for 3 hours, then every four hours. Warm other extremities. Rest and straighten or slightly bend (10°) the affected extremity for 6 hours. Inform patients about the need for frequent vitals checks and bed rest with extended limbs.	Regular extremities perfusion checks enable prompt treatment, increases blood flow, minimizing local bleeding. Bed rest and no bending enhance circulation and reduce clot risk. Aids comprehension and teamwork.
Prevent bleeding and contrast media-related tissue injury/ infection	Check vital signs as directed. Get baseline pre-cath lab values. Check the extremity's color, warmth, capillary refill, and distal pulses. Check catheterization site pressure dressing and bleeding every 30 minutes. Apply continual direct pressure one inch above the puncture site and call the doctor if bleeding occurs. Follow the six-hour bed rest directive after catheterization.	Vital sign changes may indicate internal bleeding, the first sign of medical concerns. Comparisons for post-catheterization evaluation. Regular extremities perfusion checks allow timely intervention. Keep pressure on the location to prevent bleeding/ leaking. Bed rest prevents strain and bleeding. A 45-degree head elevation and slight knee bend are appropriate.

Desirable Outcome

1. Warm and pink extremities.
2. Analogous bilateral pulses distal to the catheterization site.
3. Axillary temperature below 100°F.
4. Patient comfortability.
5. No bleeding from the puncture.
6. A normal HR and BP.

Cardiogenic Shock

Cardiogenic shock or pump failure causes reduced cardiac output, compromising heart perfusion, and inducing severe left-sided cardiac failure.

Pathophysiology

1. Disabled myocardial contractility.
2. Lung congestion due to blood pooling in the left ventricle.
3. Raised HR compensates for stroke volume loss.
4. Reduced cardiac perfusion.
5. Left-sided heart failure.
6. Myocardial hypoxia is the end outcome.

Types

1. Coronary is more common and found in 5%–10% MI. End-stage cardiomyopathy and ischemia are other causes.
2. Noncoronary occurs in conditions that compromise and strain myocardial functions, such as massive hemorrhage.

Men are more likely to get cardiogenic shock due to their higher coronary artery disease rate; thrombolytics, improved interventional methods, and better therapeutics have reduced cardiogenic shock mortality from 80%–90% to 56%–67% (Belleza, 2023).

Symptoms

Symptoms are due to impaired tissue perfusion in the skin, kidneys, and the brain.

1. Clammy skin
2. Decreased SBP by 30 mm Hg
3. Tachycardia
4. Rapid respiration
5. Oliguria
6. Confusion
7. Cyanosis

Diagnosis

Diagnoses include pulse oximetry and ABG, pulmonary artery diastolic pressure (PADP), pulmonary capillary wedge pressure (PCWP), cardiac output/cardiac index monitoring, and measurement of serum magnesium (Mg)and potassium (K). Maintain oxygen saturation at ≥ 90%. The partial pressure of carbon dioxide (PaCO2) rises with hypoxia. CVP checks assess right heart filling. PADP and PCWP reflect left-sided fluid volumes. Deficiency of Mg and K causes dysrhythmias.

Nursing Care Plan

Priorities

1. Managing low CO.
2. Monitoring vital signs and hemodynamic stability.
3. Improving gas exchange and oxygenation.

The following table shows assessment, interventions, and rationale.

Assessment	Interventions	Rationale
Decreased cardiac output	Sensorium levels Intra Arterial BP checks ECG for MI/pericardial tamponade (low voltage QRS) S3 (signifies left heart failure) and S4 (diminished ventricular compliance)	Older individuals are vulnerable to reduced perfusion to critical organs. Auscultatory BP checks may be inaccurate. Pulse pressure (systolic minus diastolic) is reduced in shock.
Optimization of oxygenation, gas exchange, and tissue perfusion.	Respiratory rate, rhythm, and depth. Consciousness levels. Cyanosis or pallor in the skin, nail beds, and mucous membranes. Airways suction for productive cough and secretions. Head-end elevation. Oxygen when needed. Mechanical ventilation preparation if this is ineffective. Fluid and drug administration per order.	Initially increased (hypercapnia and hypoxia), but with shock progression, breathing becomes shallow; patients may hyperventilate. It precedes respiratory failure. Headache and restlessness are early signs of hypoxia. Cool, pale, or bluish skin is a vasoconstrictive response to hypoxemia. Suction frees the airways. A raised head-end facilitates optimal ventilation. Fluids and drugs maintain filling pressures, CO, and cardiac workload.
Positioning of the patient	Semi-Fowler's position Position alterations every two hours.	Enhanced renal filtration and relieved pulmonary congestion. Improved breathing and reduction of pressure ulcers.
Anxiousness reduction.	Assess anxiety levels, causes, and previous coping mechanisms used.	Interventions work best when they fit the client's coping patterns.
Surgery	Prepare the patient for surgery if medical management fails.	If medicine doesn't work, surgery (coronary artery bypass) may be suggested.
Peripheral perfusion	Capillary refill Respiratory status. Accurate IV fluid amounts.	Fluid overload can decompensate the patient
Diet	Instruct the client to eat less salt.	Low-sodium diets reduce fluid and electrolyte retention.

Cardiomyopathy

The heart muscle tightens, stretches, and stiffens in Cardiomyopathy (CM), affecting its ability to pump blood. It can occur at any age and may have no known cause.

Types of Cardiomyopathy

Dilated Cardiomyopathy (DCM)

DCM is the most common type of CM. An enlarged heart impairs systolic (contraction) function.

Causes

1. Cardiotoxic agents like alcohol and cocaine
2. Genetic causes
3. CAD
4. Type 2 diabetes
5. HTN
6. MI
7. Myocarditis, HIV infections
8. Congenital heart disease
9. Pregnancy complications

Symptoms

1. Tiredness
2. Reduced exercise capacity
3. Dyspnea at rest/orthopnea(Shortness of breath on lying down is relieved by standing or sitting up)/paroxysmal nocturnal dyspnea (Waking up with shortness of breath, usually after two hours of sleep, and relieved in the upright position)

Hypertrophic Cardiomyopathy

Left ventricular wall thickening reduces the heart's blood-pumping ability. It may cause atrial fibrillation (AFib) or other arrhythmias, heart failure, and stroke. It is a major cause of sudden cardiac death in young adults.

Causes

1. Rare and familial condition.

Symptoms

1. Exertional dyspnea
2. Angina
3. Fatigue
4. Syncope

Restrictive Cardiomyopathy

This least common type of CM causes scarring/stiffening of the cardiac muscles.

Causes

1. Idiopathic
2. Endomyocardial fibrosis
3. Cancer
4. Ventricular thrombus

Symptoms

1. Edema (swelling of lower limbs/face)
2. Exercise intolerance and fatigue
3. Dyspnea

Nursing Care Plan

The following table show cardiomyopathy care plan.

Assessment	Interventions	Rationale
Intensity and uniformity of lung sounds and crackles.	Demonstrate and teach pursed-lip breathing	It slows respirations and releases trapped air and CO2 (Wagner, 2023).
Fast breathing, bounding pulses, and low oxygen saturation may indicate poor gas exchange. Cognitive impairment and restlessness can occur from insufficient brain oxygenation. Track ABGs. Hypercapnia or blood CO2 accumulation. can cause dizziness, confusion, and headaches.	IV or oral diuretics can rid the body of excess fluid. Check vitals. Give supplemental oxygen when required. Teach to seek medical help by recognizing chest pain/discomfort Breathing shortness Worsening activity tolerance Syncope or dizziness	Reducing excess fluid accumulation improves breathing and activity tolerance. Severe hypercapnia can cause dysrhythmias and respiratory failure.
Diet advice	Suggest a well-balanced diet and instruct the DASH (Dietary Approaches to Stop Hypertension) eating plan to control blood pressure.	It will prevent worsening hypertension and promote heart health.

Dysrhythmias

Correctly interpret the heart rhythm and assess the patient quickly. Examine the patient's hemodynamic response to rhythm variations. Finding the causes of dysrhythmia is vital. Fever causes tachycardias, reducing cardiac output and BP. Untreated electrolyte imbalances can cause fatal dysrhythmias.

Always evaluate and treat patients, not monitors. Dysrhythmias result from impulse creation, conduction disorders, or both. The sino-atrial (SA) node, atria, atrioventricular (AV) node, and His-Purkinje system have automatic firing cells. The *SA node (right atrium) spontaneously fires 60–100 times/minute to pace the heart.* Conduction follows the AV node, the left and right bundle His-Purkinje system, and ventricles. The heart pumps blood into circulation through rhythmic contraction and relaxation. A secondary pacemaker from another site can fire in two ways. An SA node firing slower than the secondary pacemaker may cause electrical signals to "escape." The secondary pacemaker, the AV node at 40–60 beats/minute or the His-Purkinje system at 20–40 beats/ minute, fires automatically. Secondary pacemakers can start by firing sooner than the SA node pacemaker. The atria, AV node, or ventricles may have an ectopic focus or accessory route that causes early or late "triggered" beats, causing dysrhythmia instead of sinus rhythm.

Impaired conduction and blockages, such as infarction, activate unblocked parts earlier. Uneven conduction in a unidirectional block may allow the initial impulse to reenter areas that were not excitable initially but recovered. The reentering impulse may depolarize the atria and ventricles, generating a premature beat. Continued reentrant stimulation causes tachycardia.

Dysrhythmia Types

The following are different types of dysrhythmias.

Name	Rate and rhythm	P wave	PR interval	QRS complex
Normal sinus rhythm	60–100 bpm	Normal (N)	N	N
Sinus bradycardia	< 60 bpm and regular	N	N	N
Sinus tachycardia	> 101–200 bpm, regular (R)	N	N	N
Premature atrial contraction	Usually 60–100 bpm and irregular	Abnormal shape	N	N
1st degree AV block	N and R	N	> 0.20 se	N

Name	Rate and rhythm	P wave	PR interval	QRS complex
2nd degree AV block	Type I (Mobitz I, Wenckebach heart block): Atrial beats normal and regular. Ventricular beats are slower and irregular. Type II (Mobitz II): normal and regular atrial beats, slower and regular or irregular ventricular beats.	Type I: Normal Type II: More P waves per QRS complex such as 2:1, 3:1	Type I: Progressive lengthening Type II: Normal or prolonged	Type I: Normal QRS width; blocked QRS complex Type II: Wide QRS, preceded by ≥ 2 P waves, and blocked QRS complex
3rd degree AV block	Regular atrial patterns may appear irregular as P waves are hidden in QRS complexes. Ventricular beats are 20–60/min and regular.	Normal without relation to QRS complex.	Variable	N/wide, no relation to P
Name	Rate and rhythm	P wave	PR interval	QRS complexes
Atrial flutter	Atrial rates are 200–350 bpm regular. Ventricular rates > or < 100 bpm regular/irregular	Flutter (F) waves with a sawtooth pattern are more than QRS complexes in a 2:1, 3:1, 4:1, etc., pattern	Unmeasurable	N
Atrial fibrillation	Atrial rate is 350–600 bpm with irregular ventricular > or < 100 bpm	Fibrillatory F waves	Unmeasurable	N
Premature ventricular contraction	Any rate, regular or irregular rhythm	Not seen	Unmeasurable	Distorted and wide

Name	Rate and rhythm	P wave	PR interval	QRS complex
Ventricular tachycardia	150–250 bpm; regular or irregular	Not seen	Unmeasurable	Distorted and wide
Accelerated idioventricular rhythm	40–100 bpm and regular	Not seen	Unmeasurable	Distorted and wide
Paroxysmal supraventricular tachycardia	150–220 bpm, regular	Abnormal, may be hidden in the previous T wave	N/Short (S)	N
Ventricular fibrillation	Unrecordable and irregular	Absent	Unmeasurable	Unmeasurable

Causes

1. Cardiac

   a. Valvular diseases
   b. Cardiomyopathy
   c. Conduction defects
   d. Heart failure
   e. Myocardial ischemia/infarction

2. Acid-base imbalances
3. Alcohol
4. Caffeine, tobacco
5. Connective tissue disorders
6. Drugs, antidysrhythmia drugs, stimulants, β-adrenergic blockers/toxicity
7. Electric shock
8. Electrolyte imbalances: hyperkalemia, hypocalcemia
9. Emotional crisis
10. Herbal supplements like areca nut, wahoo root bark, yerba maté
11. Hypoxia
12. Metabolic conditions: thyroid dysfunction
13. Near-drowning
14. Sepsis, shock
15. Toxins

Diagnosis

ECG tracings are diagnostic. Note the following features methodically:

1. Is the P wave upright or inverted in I, II, aVF, and V4 - V6? P is negative in aVR. Does each QRS complex have one or more P? Are there atrial fibrillatory or flutter waves?
2. Evaluate the atrial rhythm and whether or not it is regular.
3. Determine the atrial rate.
4. Measure PR interval. Is it prolonged (normal ≤ 0.11 seconds)?
5. Is the ventricular rhythm regular or irregular?
6. Determine the ventricular rate.
7. Measure the duration of the QRS complex (normal ≤ 0.12 seconds).
8. Is the ST segment isoelectric (flat), elevated, or depressed?
9. Measure the duration of the QT interval (normal ≤ 0.40 seconds for males and 0.44 seconds for females).
10. Is the T wave upright or inverted (normal: upright in leads V2–V6, inverted in aVR)?

Also, consider the following:

1. The dominant or underlying rhythm and/or dysrhythmia.
2. The clinical significance of your findings.
3. The specific treatment.

Unmonitored dysrhythmias are difficult to control. Cardiac monitoring is crucial if the patient has symptoms like chest pain. Activate emergency medical services (EMS).

Inpatient or outpatient electrophysiologic studies, Holter monitoring, event monitoring (or loop recorder), exercise treadmill testing, and signal-averaged ECGs can help diagnose dysrhythmias in hospital settings. An electrophysiologic study (EPS) can diagnose heart blockages, dysrhythmias, and syncope.

EPS can also find accessory pathways and evaluate antidysrhythmia medicines. The Holter monitor records the ECG as the patient performs daily duties. Patients keep diaries of symptoms and activities and diary entries related to ECG dysrhythmias. Only symptomatic patients use event monitors.

Smartphones store ECGs and identify atrial fibrillation. A treadmill test measures heart rhythm during exercise. Doctors analyze exercise-induced dysrhythmias, ECG abnormalities, and pharmaceutical treatment. Late potentials on the signal-averaged ECG suggest severe ventricular dysrhythmias (Bucher, n.d.).

Signs and Symptoms

1. Tachycardia/bradycardia
2. Low/high blood pressure
3. Reduced O2 saturation
4. Pain in the chest, neck, shoulder, back, jaw, or arm
5. Dizziness/fainting
6. Dyspnea
7. Extreme agitation, anxiety
8. Confusion/decreased sensorium
9. Sense of impending doom
10. Numbness/tingling
11. Weakness/extreme tiredness
12. Cold and clammy skin, pallor
13. Diminished peripheral pulse
14. Profuse sweating
15. Palpitation
16. Nausea and vomiting

Nursing Care Plan

1. Ensure the ABCs of emergency protocol: airway, breathing, and CPR (cardiopulmonary resuscitation).
2. Give Oxygen (O2) via nasal cannula or a non-rebreather mask.
3. Take baseline vitals.
4. Perform 12-lead ECG and continuous ECG monitoring.
5. Determine the underlying rate and rhythm.
6. Diagnose dysrhythmia type.
7. Make an IV access.
8. Send laboratory studies (CBC, electrolytes, etc.)

9. Ongoing monitoring includes vital signs, level of consciousness, O2 saturation, and cardiac rhythm.
10. Anticipate using antidysrhythmia drugs and analgesics.
11. Determine the necessity for intubation.
12. Prepare to start advanced cardiac life support (CPR, defibrillation, transcutaneous pacing).

Heart Failure

Heart failure (HF), or Congestive Heart Failure (CHF), occurs when the heart fails to pump blood effectively to the rest of the body. It can be classified as follows.

Left heart failure (LVF): The left ventricle loses contractility (systolic HF) or stiffens and cannot relax and fill with blood between beats (diastolic HF).

Right ventricular failure (RVF) usually follows LVF. Blood pools in the veins due to right ventricle dysfunction, producing CHF. Possible causes include heart attack, chronic pulmonary disease, valve malfunction, etc. Commonly, HF affects both hearts or biventricular failure.

HF can be acute or chronic. Acute cardiac failure is sudden with severe initial symptoms. With effective therapy, recovery is quick. Heart attacks and decompensated chronic HF can cause acute heart failure with worsening symptoms, including shortness of breath. It requires hospitalization. Chronic heart failure symptoms begin slowly and worsen.

The ejection fraction describes the strength and ability of the heart's chambers to empty with each contraction (beat). Echocardiography measures it.

Reduction of the main pumping chamber's pumping ability is heart failure with reduced ejection fraction (HFrEF). Conversely, a primary diastolic relaxation problem impairs filling, which is heart failure with preserved ejection fraction (HFpEF). These problems often overlap with both reduced emptying and filling.

Preload is the initial stretching of the myocardium before contraction. It is related to ventricular filling. Afterload is the force against which the heart must contract to eject the blood. Afterload falls with the lowering of aortic pressure and systemic vascular resistance through vasodilation (e.g., antihypertensives).

Causes

1. CAD
2. MI
3. Hypertension
4. Valvular disease
5. Myocarditis
6. Congenital heart defects
7. Cardiac dysrhythmias
8. Poorly managed chronic conditions such as diabetes mellitus, HIV, hyper/hypothyroidism, lung diseases

Stage of Heart Failure Determination

Staging depends on the extent of activity intolerance.

1. Class I: Normal physical activity.
2. Class II: ADL without difficulty, but shortness of breath and some fatigue on exertion.
3. Class III: ADL is associated with fatigue, palpitations, or dyspnea.
4. Class IV: Dyspnea at rest.

Risk Factors

Non-modifiable risk factors are unchanged. They include

1. Age (> 65)
2. Gender (twice as common in males)
3. Family history (first-degree female relative with heart disease < 65 years or a first-degree male relative with heart disease < 55 years)

4. Race/ethnicity (more common in African Americans and Latinos than in Caucasians)

Modifiable risk factors are remediable and include

1. Hypertension
2. Hypercholesterolemia/CAD
3. Diabetes
4. Valvular heart diseases
5. Tobacco
6. Obesity
7. Lack of physical activity
8. Poor dietary habits
9. Stress/inadequate sleep
10. Alcohol use
11. Some medications

    a. Nonsteroidal anti-inflammatory drugs (NSAIDs)
    b. Some diabetes medications
    c. Antihypertensive medications (some calcium channel blockers)
    d. Medications for cancer, blood disorders, psychiatry, etc.

12. Bacterial and viral infections, such as:

    a. Influenza
    b. Pneumonia
    c. Urinary tract infections
    d. Bacteremia
    e. Covid-19
    f. HIV

Nursing Care Plan

The following table shows nursing assessment, diagnosis, and desired outcomes.

Assessment	Diagnosis	Desired Outcome
Excess fluid accumulation	Dyspnea, weight gain, edema, neck vein distention, crackles in lungs, cough, tachycardia, and S3 heart sound	Patients will maintain steady fluid volume. They will express fluid overload symptoms and know fluid limits.
Assessment	**Interventions**	**Rationale**
Reduced cardiac output	Palpitations Dysrhythmias Dyspnea/Orthopnea Neck vein distention/ edema Central venous pressure changes Diminished peripheral pulses and urine	Normal vital signs, cardiac output, and renal perfusion indicate hemodynamic stability. Activities will lower cardiac workload. The patient will not mention chest discomfort or breathlessness.
Reduced cardiac tissue perfusion	Hypotension Increased CVP/pulmonary artery pressure (PAP) Tachycardia Dysrhythmia EF < 40%	Patients will have normal pulse and rhythm. Patients will have > 40% ejection fraction. Patients will have palpable peripheral pulses.
Assess patient feedback and degree of debility regarding activity intolerance and cardiopulmonary response to activity, which involves heart rate, oxygen saturation, and cardiac rhythm during activity.	Weakness Dyspnea Sluggishness Vital sign changes to activity Exertional chest pain	Patients will do limited activity to avoid cardiac stress. Immobility increases risks for skin breakdown, deep vein thrombosis (DVT), and pneumonia. Patients will rest between works to complete ADLs. Patients will have vital signs and cardiac rhythm within normal limits during activities.

Interventions

Intervention	Rationale
Improve perfusion: administer drugs like angiotensin-converting enzyme (ACE) inhibitors and angiotensin II receptor blockers (ARBs) Administer beta blockers Diuretics Potassium-sparing diuretics IV inotropes and digoxin (monitor toxicity levels)	Improve blood flow by relaxing the blood vessels, reducing BP and cardiac strain. Reduce the HR and BP. Remove excess fluid from the body. Manage systolic HF Improve the effectiveness of heart muscles
Manage underlying conditions per order.	Removal of causative factors improves heart functions.
Interventions	Rationale
Surgical interventions: prepare the patient for procedures like CABG/ valvular replacement or repair/cardiac resynchronization therapy (CRT)/ heart transplant. CRT corrects the electrical signals in arrhythmias using a biventricular pacemaker.	Surgery may be required.
Cardiac rehabilitation: improve activity tolerance gradually. Implantable cardioverter-defibrillators (ICDs) track the heart rhythm to maintain a regular heart rate if an arrhythmia develops. Emphasize lifestyle adjustments. Instruct the patient to contact the healthcare team if their weight gain is> 1kg overnight or 2.3kg/week. Limit sodium (salt) intake to prevent water retention.	Collaborate with the team to meet the health needs of the patient. Lifestyle modification improves cardiac strength and checks complications. Stress compromises cardiac muscle function. Excess fluid accumulation increases the preload. Follow-ups prevent recurrences and complications. Using medical IDs alert others to a patient's condition during an emergency.

Hypertension (HTN)

1. Normal Blood Pressure is < 120/80
2. Prehypertension is 120–139/80-89
3. Stage 1 Hypertension is 140–159/90-99
4. Stage 2 Hypertension is > 160/100

Hypertension increases the risk of heart failure, stroke, and artery hardening by making the heart work harder to pump blood. Risks for hypertension include:

1. Overweight or obesity
2. Smoking
3. Genetics/family history
4. A salty diet
5. Drinking more than 1-2 alcoholic drinks daily
6. Stress
7. Old age
8. Inactivity
9. Obstructive sleep apnea
10. Kidney disease
11. Thyroid disorders

It is crucial to know the North American Nursing Diagnosis Association (NANDA) definition, signs of evidence, desired goal, and nurse actions for each hypertension nursing diagnosis (Douglas, n.d.).

The following table describes nursing activities concerning HTN.

NANDA definition	Evidence	Desired outcome	Intervention
The heart pumps too little blood to meet metabolic needs	This is a preventive diagnosis	The patient can Control heart rhythm and pace. ControlBP. Do activities to reduce BP and cardiac burden.	Check the patient's lab data (cardiac indicators, blood cell count, electrolytes, ABGs, etc.) for contributory factors. Record both arm and thigh blood pressure. Check breath sounds and cardiac rhythm. Examine the patient's skin color, temperature, and capillary refill time. Encourage the patient to cut sodium.

NANDA definition	Evidence	Desired outcome	Intervention
Pain (typically headaches) is an experience or anticipation of painful sensory and emotional sensations due to existing or potential tissue injury. Sudden/slow onset Mild to severe intensity Predictable end Duration.	Head throbbing usually upon awakening. Appetite changes. Patients experience neck stiffness, impaired vision, disorientation, nausea, and vomiting.	The patient reports being headache and pain-free.	Assess pain severity, location, and duration. Record the patient's pain tolerance and drug use. Promote rest and relaxation, including neck and back massages, cool forehead clothes, and avoiding strong lighting. Restrict patient mobility. Assess analgesic needs.
Activity intolerance, physical or mental.	Weak or tired patient. Activities cause abnormal heart rate. Dyspnea from exercise. ECG indicating ischemia or dysrhythmias.	Patient does desired actions. Improves activity tolerance using identified methods. Reports increased activity tolerance. Shows less intolerance.	List each fatigue-prone element (age/ disease). Check the patient's activity intolerance and timing. Check the patient's pulse, heart rate, chest pain, dizziness, and fatigue. Show energy-saving activities.
Coping issues are defined as an inability to assess stressors, choose appropriate responses, or employ existing resources.	Patients request assistance suggesting coping inability. Patients show stress, anger, anxiety, and depression. Features of overeating, lack of appetite, and smoking/ alcohol abuse are present.	Patients acknowledge weak coping mechanisms and coping skills. Patients avoid/change unpleasant situations. Patients cope well.	Explore what the patient struggles with. Evaluate the patient's coping skills and suggest changes. Help the patient identify and manage stressors. Develop a treatment plan with the patient and encourage cooperation. Help the patient identify and plan lifestyle modifications. Encourage the patient to assess life objectives and priorities.

NANDA definition	Evidence	Desired outcome	Intervention
Impaired nutrition is described as taking more nutrients than needed.	Patients weigh 10%–20% more than optimal for their height and shape. Abnormal eating habits.	The patient understands the association between obesity and hypertension. Maintains a good exercise routine. Shows diet choices and changes in quantities to lose weight.	Assess and discuss the patient's understanding of hypertension and obesity. Determine the patient's weight loss objective. Create a manageable fitness routine for the patient. Make realistic nutrition plans with dietitians.
Knowledge deficit is a lack of topic-specific cognitive information.	Sharing the issue. Patients require more/don't understand information. Patients disregard orders. Patients seem agitated or disturbed about their condition and therapy.	Patients can relate to hypertension management and treatment. Patients use prescribed medications correctly and understand side effects.	Assess learning readiness and barriers. Include the partners if feasible. Explain hypertension, how it affects the body and treatment. Control BP rather than normalizing it.

Educate HTN patients on hypertension management adjustments, the necessity of weight stability, low-calorie, low-sodium diets, and HTN resources.

Hypertensive Crisis

Sudden, significant blood pressure increases of 180/120 mm Hg or higher is called a hypertensive crisis—a medical emergency that can cause a heart attack or stroke.

Nursing Care Plan

Assessment

1. Headache
2. Visual blurring
3. Dyspnea
4. Chest pain
5. Dizzy
6. Anxiety
7. Sense of doom

Interventions

1. Frequently monitor BP.
2. Administer prescribed antihypertensive medications to maintain the target BP set by the physician.
3. Insert two large-bore IVs.
4. Administer oxygen for low oxygen saturation < 94%.
5. Restrict fluid intake in patients with heart failure.
6. Monitor ECG for indications of a heart attack/dysrhythmias.
7. Check chest X-rays to assess if the patient has heart failure signs.
8. Listen for heart murmurs (HF) and lungs for rales and crackles (CHF).
9. Check for peripheral edema (HF).
10. Check renal function (urea and creatinine) and electrolyte levels (renal perfusion and kidney failure).
11. Ensure rest in a semi-Fowler position; keep a quiet room.
12. Post-crisis, train the patient on stress reduction techniques (yoga, deep breathing exercises, etc.).
13. Instruct DASH diet, exercise, and healthy eating practices (adequate and timely meals).
14. Teach the necessity of taking regular antihypertensive medications and BP checks.
15. Seek team help

    a. Altered level of consciousness (LOC)/Unresponsive
    b. BP > 200/100 despite treatment.

Desired Outcome

Although short-term success is possible, patient dropout and pharmacological adjustments have long-term effects. Educate patients about hypertension to reduce morbidity and mortality from untreated hypertension.

Care Coordination

Hypertensive emergencies come to the ER. At least 50% of patients with hypertension remain noncompliant with their medications despite receiving education about disease seriousness (Alley et al., 2023).

Minimally-Invasive Cardiac Surgery (Non-Sternal Approach)

Minimally invasive heart surgery requires chest incisions. The surgeon can access the heart between the ribs. Unlike open-heart surgery, the breastbone remains intact.

Applications

1. Repairing/replacing valvular defects
2. Atrioventricular septal defect (ASD) surgery
3. Maze procedure in atrial fibrillation
4. Removing tumors from the heart

In comparison to open-heart surgery, the benefits are:

1. Minimal blood loss
2. Lower infection rates
3. Decreased pain
4. Reduced ventilation time
5. Shorter hospital stays
6. A faster recovery
7. Smaller scars

Patient Advice

Patients can bring the following items to the hospital:

1. Glasses, hearing aids, dentures
2. Personal care goods like toothbrushes, combs, razors, etc
3. Comfortable loose clothing
4. Copy of advance directive
5. Portable music players and reading material
6. Medication list and information on drug allergy

During Surgery

Ensure the patient does not wear the following items during surgery:

1. Contact lenses
2. Dentures
3. Eyeglasses
4. Jewelry
5. Nail polish

Type

Surgery frequently involves a heart-lung bypass machine, which circulates blood during surgery.

1. Robotic heart surgery: The surgeon controls the arms using a nearby computer. A magnified 3D heart image on a video monitor informs the surgeon. The robotic arms move with the surgeon's arms and wrists to perform surgery. Robotic arms carry surgical tools, replaced by the operating team as needed.
2. Thoracoscopic or mini-thoracotomy surgery: Surgeons approach the heart with small chest rib incisions. They use a small video camera to see inside the body through an incision.

Post-Op Nursing Care

Minimally invasive heart surgery usually requires one night in the ICU. Administer and monitor the following per order:

1. Intravenous fluids and medications
2. Bladder/chest fluid and blood drain tubes
3. Oxygen through face masks or nasal cannulas

The ICU stay is followed by recovery in the ward. The type of surgery and health determine the duration of the hospital stay. The following actions are crucial during this time:

1. Surveillance for signs of infection.
2. Assessment of vitals.
3. Pain medication administration as necessary.
4. Gradual patient ambulation.
5. Deep breathing techniques and coughing to clear the lungs.
6. Removal of drainage tubes.

Post-surgery health checks are frequently required, and tests can assess heart function. The heart rehabilitation program includes a customized fitness and education program to strengthen the patient after surgery. Supervised exercise, emotional support, and heart-healthy lifestyle teaching are part of cardiac rehabilitation.

Valvular Heart Disease

The heart has four valves:

1. The mitral valve between the left atrium and left ventricle.
2. The tricuspid valve between the right atrium and right ventricle.
3. The pulmonary valve.
4. The aortic valve.

Valvular defects are of two types: stenosis and regurgitation. Stenosis, or narrowing of the valve orifice, increases cardiac strain. Valvular regurgitations allow blood to flow back into the heart as the valve leaflets do not seal completely on closure.

Types and Causes

1. Regurgitation

    a. Congenital defects
    b. Acute rheumatic carditis
    c. Hypertension
    d. Dilated cardiomyopathy
    e. Traumatic valve rupture
    f. Senile degeneration
    g. Syphilitic aortitis
    h. Mitral valve prolapse
    i. Aortic aneurysm

2. Stenosis

    a. Congenital defects
    b. Rheumatic heart
    c. Senile degeneration
    d. Carcinoid tumors

Symptoms and Signs

1. Breathing difficulty
2. Dizziness
3. Wheeze/heavy cough
4. Exertional fatigue
5. Palpitations/mild chest pain
6. Fever (infective etiology)
7. Rapid weight gain (HF)
8. Swelling of the ankles/feet/abdomen.

Diagnosis

1. ECG, echocardiogram and Radionuclide scans
2. Stress testing
3. Angiogram

Nursing Care Plan

Assessment	Diagnosis	Intervention
Mental status	Restlessness Severe anxiety Confusion	Improve perfusion.
Assessment	Diagnosis	Interventions
Heart sounds	Note gallops, S3, S4	Inform the doctor.
Emergencies	Signs of HF/dysrhythmias	Check vitals
Cardiac output	Diminished peripheral pulse Cold, clammy skin Poor appetite Increased/decreased weight	Check peripheral pulses manually for rate and rhythm Monitor intake output and daily weight Administer stool softeners to reduce cardiac strain.
Lung	Dyspnea/orthopnea	Check respiration rate, distress, and lung sound. Keep the patient in semi- to high-Fowler's position. Administer O2 per order.
Treat underlying acute conditions	Monitor CVP, PAP, and right atrial pressure (RAP).	Administer prescribed medications and observe response, side effects, and toxicity.

Peripheral Vascular Diseases

Causes

1. Functional

    a. Stress

    b. Smoking

    c. Cold temperature

    d. Operating machinery or tools

2. Drugs
3. Structural changes in blood vessels due to aging (> 50), overweight, history of heart disease/stroke, kidney disease/hemodialysis.

Symptoms and Signs

1. Weak leg and foot pulses
2. Feet and legs may have brittle, thin, or glossy skin
3. Lowered skin temperature
4. Gangrene
5. Impotence
6. Leg-specific hair loss
7. Muscle weakness, numbness, and heaviness
8. Pressure-point wounds that don't heal
9. Leg pallor when elevated
10. Aching or burning toes at rest
11. Restricted mobility
12. Extremities discolored red to blue
13. Thickened toenails
14. Obstructed arteries cause severe agony

Risk Factors

1. Sedentary habits
2. Poor dietary habits
3. Smoking
4. Drug use
5. Elevated BP

6. Increased cholesterol
7. Diabetes

Diagnosis

1. Doppler ultrasound
2. Ankle-Brachial index is low
3. Magnetic resonance angiography
4. Angiography/CT angiography

Nursing Care Plan

NANDA description	Evidence	Desired outcome	Interventions
Impaired skin integrity related to immobility.	Local redness Ulcerations/ eczema. Elevated temperature. Feeling unwell.	The patient will describe changes in tissue impairment and discomfort. The patient will comprehend tissue healing and damage prevention. The wounds shrink, and granulated tissues grow.	Assess wound and tissue damage. Check for redness, edema, and pallor. Check the temperature for infections. Promote skincare. When necessary, use antibiotics. Check for DVT. Do not scratch wound.

NANDA description	Evidence	Desired outcome	Interventions
Acute Pain	Facial distortion, guarding of body parts, and changes in the vital signs.	The patient will relax using diversions and skills. The patient will report satisfactory pain control. Vital signs will be normal.	Assess the patient's vital signs and pain scale. Ask about past pain medications, efficacy, duration, and adverse effects or allergies. Massage, heat and cold application, acupressure, contralateral stimulation, and therapeutic exercise may reduce pain. Administer medication as directed. Assess the patient's response to interventions and management.
Fatigue	Lethargy, lack of interest in surroundings, and inability to participate in ADLs.	The patient will be more active and energetic. Patients' fatigue causes will be better understood. The patient will discuss energy conservation. Interventions and exercises will assist the patient in overcoming weariness.	Question the patient about exhaustion, its severity, and its treatments. Physical illness, mental stress, depression, prescription side effects, sleeping pattern disorders, and poor diet can induce fatigue. Assess the patient's daily task performance. Evaluate the patient's diet, energy, and metabolic needs. Check the patient's fatigue, anxiety, and depression. Instruct adequate rest.
Tissue perfusion	Cool skin, hair loss, and weak pulse.	Development of warm skin and strong pulse.	Check limb color, temperature and feel.

Nursing Procedures

Ablation

Cardiac ablation means destroying specific cardiac cells, causing or routing tachy-dysrhythmias. Indications include:

1. Recurrent atrial dysrhythmia
2. AFib
3. Ventricular tachycardia unresponsive to therapy
4. Wolff-Parkinson-White syndrome

High-frequency, low-energy sound waves are passed through a catheter to produce thermal ablation of specific tissues, causing dysrhythmia and less trauma to the surrounding heart tissue than cryoablation/electrical ablation.

The procedure requires defibrillation pads, an automatic BP cuff, a pulse oximeter, and a urinary catheter. Post-op care is the same as electrophysiology studies, with more surveillance during the sedation period.

Arterial Closure Devices

Vascular access closure devices are used for arterial procedures with 6F catheters or bigger at the common femoral artery entry sites. A proceduralist (vascular surgeon), first assistant (resident, fellow, cath lab technician, physician assistant), radiology technician, and nursing staff perform the procedure. Depending on the operation, the anesthesiologist may be present.

The procedure requires

1. Sterile drapes
2. Local anesthetic
3. Hemostat
4. Scalpel
5. Micropuncture kit for percutaneous common femoral artery approach

6. Ultrasound machine
7. A .035 wire (stiff angled guidewire or Bentson wire) and contrast
8. A 5F/6F short sheath catheter
9. A fluoroscopic imaging system (C-arm)
10. Lead shielding, heparinized saline
11. Heparin
12. Vascular access closure device

The micropuncture is below the inguinal ligament and superior femoral head and away from calcified, superficial, and deep arteries. A hemostat spreads tissues to access the arterial level. The micropuncture wire is removed after the 4F catheter is inserted.

A femoral angiogram is used to check the access site and vascular compatibility for the closure device (especially size and arterial plaque) to prevent perforation or dissection. Monitor the patient for 30–120 minutes to prevent hemorrhage.

Arterial/Venous Sheaths

Cardiologists and vascular surgeons conduct endovascular treatments that may leave arterial or venous sheaths in place. Removing the sheath may increase patient ease and reduce bed rest, improving patient outcomes. However, sheath removal is risky and requires proper nursing training.

After sheath removal, manual compression (alone or with a hemostasis pad), mechanical compression, collagen plug, and percutaneous suture-mediated closure devices prevent bleeding. Due to muscle fatigue and injury, healthcare workers applying manual compression may develop carpal tunnel syndrome. Mechanical compression prevents hematomas and other issues.

Instruments

1. Gloves
2. Gown
3. Goggles/face shield with mask

4. ECG monitor
5. BP monitor
6. Permanent marker
7. Antiseptic solution (chlorhexidine-based)
8. Sterile gauze and gloves
9. Suture removal kit
10. Hypoallergenic tape
11. Linen-saver pad
12. Sterile saline solution (for noninvasive hemostasis pad)
13. Transparent dressing (for noninvasive hemostasis pad)
14. Mechanical compression device

Before the Procedure

1. Clean hands.
2. Check the doctor's sheath removal order.
3. According to facility regulations, the patient's identity must be verified with two identifiers.

Preparation

1. Explain the method to lessen patient anxiety and improve participation. Include activity restrictions, pressure-related discomfort, and post-procedure effects.
2. To ensure hemostasis, monitor the patient's platelet count, prothrombin time (PT), PTT, complete blood count, International Normalized Ratio (INR), and activated clotting time before sheath removal.
3. Set a baseline using vital signs and ECG. For hemostasis, systolic blood pressure should be under 150 mm Hg.
4. Assess neurovascular state in the extremity distal to sheath insertion.
5. Use a permanent marker to locate pulses distal to the sheath insertion location.
6. Give an analgesic 20–30 minutes before the surgery for patient comfort.
7. Ensure the patient has a patent IV catheter for emergency fluids or drugs.
8. Place the patient with the head of the bed flat to encourage hemostasis.

9. To keep bed linen clean and to store the sheath after removal, insert the linen-saver pad underneath the injured extremity.
10. Place a mechanical compression device under the patient before sheath removal.
11. If the sheath is sutured, open the suture removal kit without contamination.
12. Complete the hand hygiene method and use goggles, masks, gloves, and gowns for the procedure.

Cardiac Catheterization

Cardiac catheterization is passing a catheter into the heart to measure heart chamber pressure and flow, obtain blood samples, and record contrast ventriculography, coronary arteriography, or angiography images.

The left heart catheterization checks coronary artery patency, left ventricular function, and valvular functions. The right heart catheterization checks tricuspid and pulmonic valve performance and PAP.

Pre-Procedure

1. Explain the procedure to the patient.
2. Tell them to limit fluids for six hours before the test.
3. Inform them the procedure takes one to two hours and that they will remain conscious during the surgery.
4. Ask the patient to urinate before the surgery.
5. Check for allergies to drugs or diagnostic contrast media. Discontinue anticoagulants as directed.

Post-Procedure

1. Monitor heart rate, rhythm, respiration, pulse, and blood pressure.
2. Monitor vitals every 15 minutes for 2 hours after the procedure, then every 30 minutes, then every hour.

3. Check for hematoma or blood loss at the insertion site. Controlling bleeding may require further compression.
4. Monitor every four hours in the absence of immediate complications. Check vital signs frequently and notify the doctor if unstable.
5. Assess color, skin temperature, and peripheral pulse below the puncture.
6. Force eight hours of bed rest. Keep the patient's leg extended for eight hours after femoral catheter insertion.
7. Consult the practitioner about restarting drugs withheld before the test.
8. Use prescription painkillers.
9. Schedule a posttest ECG to check for myocardial damage.

Defibrillation

Defibrillation involves passing a high-voltage electric current through electrodes on the chest wall. Proper electrode insertion places the cardiac axis between current sources (defibrillator paddles). Electric current is randomly passed because dysrhythmias are chaotic with no coordinated ventricular response. Emergent defibrillation stops ventricular fibrillation and pulseless ventricular tachycardia and restores cardiac output.

Equipment

1. Defibrillator
2. Conductive medium-defibrillator pads
3. Cardiac monitor with recorder
4. Emergency cart and medications
5. Emergency pacing equipment

Procedure

1. Check ECG for V-fib or V-tach and clinical status. Check for pulselessness. Call for aid and CPR until the defibrillator and crash cart arrive.
2. Prepare for defibrillation
3. Assess state. Establish an airway and start CPR if a second person gets the defibrillator.

4. Power "ON." The default is 200 joules.
5. Choose adult, pediatric, or internal paddles.
6. Apply conductive agent to patient and paddles.
7. The defibrillator must be in an asynchronous mode.
8. Turn on the ECG recorder for continuous printing.
9. Set one paddle at the heart's apex left of the nipple in the midaxillary line. Apply 25 pounds per square inch of pressure to the other paddle below the right clavicle to the right of the sternum.
10. Press "CHARGE" on the front/Apex paddle. Wait until it is fully charged when the indicator stops flashing.
11. Announce "ALL CLEAR" and visually ensure that all personnel are away from bed, patient, and equipment.
12. Check rhythm immediately before discharge.
13. Maintain pressure on both buttons until the electrical current arrives. Maintain 25 lbs/in2.
14. Dysrhythmia conversion assessment: If there is no response, repeat the procedures thrice after charging the paddles to 300 joules. If the third effort fails, start CPR, Advanced Cardiac Life Support (ACLS), intubation, and IV access. To prevent decompensation, assess patient status and causation.
15. Discard supplies, clean the defibrillator and paddles, and wash hands.
16. Record procedure in the patient record or cardiac arrest flowsheet.

Precautions

1. Administer supplemental oxygen.
2. Protect caregivers from flowing electric current.
3. Check ECG rhythm if it needs defibrillation.
4. Premature release may prevent energy discharge.
5. Reassess if the rhythm changed.
6. Immediate action improves cardiac muscle depolarization. The second shock reduces transthoracic resistance by 8%.
7. Immediate action improves cardiac muscle depolarization; the "stacked shocks" sequence is crucial, and delays are harmful.

Cardioversion

Cardioversion stops arrhythmias by depolarizing tissue with a synchronized shock in a reentrant circuit. According to Knight, cardioversion involves a synchronized energy supply to the QRS Complex, while defibrillation involves random shocks during the cardiac cycle (Knight, 2015). Indications include atrial flutter, atrial fibrillation, ventricular tachycardia, and ventricular fibrillation.

Procedure

1. An immediate family member's contact number must be on the permission form for informed consent.
2. Check electrolytes: K > 4 and Mg > 2; replace if low.
3. If on warfarin, maintain therapeutic INR levels (2.0–3.0) for four weeks; new oral anticoagulants (NOACs) must be continued for four weeks.
4. Ensure proper sedation to prevent aspiration.
5. Keep the suction apparatus within reach.
6. Confirm arrhythmia duration if anticoagulated incorrectly; proceed with direct current cardioversion (DCCV) if < 48 hours.
7. If the arrhythmia persists beyond 48 hours, transesophageal echocardiography (TEE) is necessary to rule out left atrial/left atrial appendage thrombus. If TEE is negative, proceed with DCCV.
8. Defibrillation success depends on the type of arrhythmia and the patient's clinical condition.

Steps

1. Verify informed consent for operation, anesthesia, and TEE (if needed).
2. Electrode placement
3. SYNC defibrillator
4. Time out
5. Appropriate anesthetic sedation
6. Select necessary Joules: Atrial Flutter: 100 J, Afib: 200 J, starting at the physician's discretion
7. Charge, Clear, Shock!

Post-Procedure

1. Patients who are awake, attentive, focused, and able to swallow can return home.
2. A relative or friend should drive owing to anesthetic residuals. Sedated patients must not drive for 24 hours.
3. An emollient lotion may be applied for local skin irritation.
4. Advise continuing anticoagulation pills for the next four weeks; other medications are per the cardiologist's advice.
5. Resume tolerated activities; no driving for 24 hours.
6. Keep appointments with doctors as scheduled.
7. Encourage adequate hydration and compliance with medication, diet, and exercises for adequate BP management.

Pacemakers

The pacemaker's primary function is maintaining a healthy heart rate to maintain blood pressure and organ perfusion. It sends an electrical signal through lead wires to depolarize and contract the heart muscle. Its parts are a pulse generator battery/brain (pacemaker regulation) and electrode-end lead cables. Check the pulse generator rate against the prescribed rate.

Pacing can be asynchronous or on-demand. Demand pacing paces on patient requirements, sensing cardiac impulses. In asynchronous pacing mode, the pacemaker fires at a predetermined rate regardless of cardiac impulses.

Dysrhythmias may require *temporary pacing* (*three days*) until the patient's rhythm stabilizes or a permanent pacemaker is inserted. *Permanent pacemakers* for various bradycardia arrhythmias require a short surgical procedure under local anesthesia.

Types

1. Transcutaneous is used for unstable rhythms in emergency situations.
2. Transvenous pacemakers stabilize arrhythmias.
3. Epicardial, the most common method, requires an open thoracotomy.

4. Transesophageal: The electrode passes through the nose or is swallowed as a pill-electrode. It is used in atrial pacing in sinus bradycardia, supraventricular tachycardia, or for diagnostic studies.

Priorities

1. Inspect the system for proper functioning.
2. Retain electrical safety.
3. Watch for complications at the insertion site.
4. Evaluate patient protection and ease.
5. Educate the patient on

    a. Reasons for pacemaker
    b. The anticipated problems
    c. Eight hours of fasting before the procedure

Preparation

1. Obtain baseline 12-lead ECG, bleeding function, and other blood work.
2. Make an IV access for fluids, sedation, and emergency drugs.
3. Check vitals, peripheral pulses, and heart/lung sounds.
4. Assess patient anxiety, listen, reassure, and sedate as needed.
5. Prepare the generator access site by shaving and cleaning.
6. Keep the field clean.
7. Keep a heart monitor on during the procedure.

Post-Surgery Observation

1. Assess dyspnea, low BP, chest discomfort, and rapid HR, suggesting complications like

    a. Pneumothorax (collapsed lung)
    b. Hemothorax (blood in the pleural cavity)
    c. Pacemaker lead perforation

    d. Cardiac tamponade (fluid buildup pressure on the heart)

2. Watch for lead dislodgement: ECG abnormalities/diaphragm hiccups.
3. Watch for ECG sensing/capture/pacing issues. Move away from the electrical device or turn off equipment that may cause pacemaker interference.
4. Administer painkillers as needed.
5. Check the insertion site for infection and bleeding.
6. Give ice packs to reduce discomfort and swelling for six hours.
7. Ensure bed rest for 12 hours.
8. Restrain the arm for 12–24 hours. After 24 hours, help restore movement with gentle ROM exercises thrice daily.
9. Avoid aspirin and heparin for 48 hours.
10. On discharge

    a. Avoid watering the place for three days.
    b. Limit arm and shoulder activity and cover the incision with a loose cloth for two weeks.
    c. Avoid lifting and contact sports for two months.
    d. Consult doctors if weariness, palpitations, or symptoms return (may indicate pacemaker malfunction or battery depletion).
    e. Take radial pulse daily on waking; contact a doctor if rates exceed programmed rates.
    f. Always carry pacemaker information and a MedicAlert bracelet (pacemakers trigger airport security alarms).

A pacemaker with an implanted cardioverter-defibrillator (ICD) can monitor heart activity and automatically countershock dysrhythmias that do not respond to antidysrhythmic medication.

Percutaneous Coronary Intervention (PCI)

Percutaneous coronary intervention (PCI) is a set of minimally invasive procedures intended to open blocked coronary arteries. Restoring blood flow can relieve symptoms like chest discomfort and shortness of breath.

A tiny incision is made in the wrist or upper thigh, and a catheter is threaded through a main artery to reach the blocked vessel. PCI types include basic balloon angioplasty, angioplasty with a stent as an element of balloon angioplasty, rotational atherectomy to remove calcified plaque, and Impella-supported PCI to maintain critical organs' blood flow in severe heart disease.

Patient Information

1. The procedure occurs under sedation and local anesthetic.
2. During the procedure, the patient will have an IV line, electrodes to monitor the heart, and a pulse oximeter.
3. A PCI may last one to three hours.
4. A contrast dye identifies the blockage, helping doctors determine the suitable PCI type.
5. For groin catheters, the patient must lie flat on their back with bent legs for several hours. Those with arm catheters will have their legs lifted on cushions and straightened with a stabilizing board.
6. The patient is moved to a recovery room for two to six hours of observation.
7. Pain medications are given if necessary.
8. Oral fluids help flush the contrast dye from the body.
9. Patients can be discharged on the same or the next day, depending on procedural ease. Self-driving is restricted for 24 hours following the procedure.
10. Shower after 24 to 48 hours; avoid lifting and pulling with the wrist for five days (playing golf; household chores), and do a five-days-a-week moderate-intensity activity (walking or swimming) after a week. Use cardiac rehab when suggested.
11. Consult doctors for

    a. Elevated pain
    b. Inflammation
    c. Bleeding/discharge from the operation site
    d. Fever/chills

Transesophageal Echocardiogram (TEE)

TEE employs ultrasonography to visualize the ascending aorta, upper heart chambers, and valves. A small tube connected to the echo transducer passes through the mouth, throat, and esophagus near the upper heart chambers, obtaining clearer images than normal echocardiograms. Ask the patient to avoid alcohol for a few days before the day procedure under a sedative. Avoid food or drinks four to six hours before the procedure. Someone should drive the patient home. During the procedure:

1. An anesthetic spray is used to numb the throat and reduce the gag reflex.
2. An IV line is made.
3. An ECG machine records the heartbeat. A small, flexible probe is passed through the mouth and throat as swallowing movements are made.
4. The probe, IV, and electrodes are removed after the procedure; the patient is monitored until they wake up. A sore throat can be present for 24-48 hours.

Monitoring Hemodynamic Status

Understanding hemodynamics helps you comprehend cardiac output, the stroke volume pumped by the heart, and the factors that affect it, such as variabilities in the normal HR, preload, afterload, and cardiac contractility.

The blood pressure and the mean arterial pressure depend on the resistance to the blood flow within the body's circulatory system. The resistance to blood flow depends on the blood viscosity, arterial width, and the vessel's length, calculated with the Hagen Poiseuille equation. Atherosclerosis and plaque buildup impede blood flow, increase resistance, and raise BP.

The normal hemodynamic values are:

1. Cardiac output: 4–7 L/min
2. CVP: 1–8 mm Hg
3. PAP systolic: 15–26 mm Hg
4. PAP diastolic: 5–15 mm Hg

5. PAP (wedge): 4–12 mm Hg
6. Pulmonary artery mean: 9–16 mm Hg
7. Pulmonary artery end diastolic: 4–14 mm Hg
8. Pulmonary artery occlusion mean: 2–12 mm Hg
9. Pulmonary artery peak systolic: 15–30 mm Hg
10. Right ventricle peak systolic: 15–30 mm Hg
11. Right ventricle end-diastolic: 0–8 mm Hg
12. Left ventricle peak systolic: 90–140 mm Hg
13. Left ventricle end-diastolic: 5–12 mm Hg
14. Left atrium mean: 2–12 mm Hg
15. Left atrium A Wave: 4–16 mm Hg
16. Left atrium V Wave: 6–12 mm Hg
17. Right atrium pressure: 0–8 mm Hg
18. Brachial artery mean: 70–150 mm Hg
19. Brachial artery peak systolic: 90–140 mm Hg
20. Brachial artery end diastolic: 60–90 mm Hg
21. Mixed venous oxygen saturation: 60%–80%

Critical nursing tasks include hemodynamic monitoring of arterial lines, pulmonary artery catheters, their proximal and distal lumen, balloon inflation port, and pulse oximeters.

Decreasing cardiac output reduces exercise tolerance with exhaustion and weakness. Falls may occur due to weakness, weariness, confusion, and other mental issues.

Recognizing the specific signs, symptoms, and ECG rhythm and knowing medical and nursing interventions and emergency care using CPR and ACLS protocols is crucial. *Nurses may monitor, assess, intervene, document, and report telemetry ECG.*

Pacemaker-related knowledge is insertion, asepsis, client care, monitoring during and after this invasive process, mechanical problems, and battery failures.

Nurses must monitor vessel puncture during placement, catheter breakage and migration, arterial hemorrhage, and infection.

Contraindications for the arterial line include severe burns at the insertion site, impaired circulation, pulselessness, Buerger's disease, and Raynaud syndrome. Other relative contraindications are atherosclerosis, a clotting disorder, impaired circulation, scar tissue near the site, and a synthetic graft.

NANDA describes altered and ineffective tissue perfusion as oxygen reduction failing to nourish tissues at the capillary level.

1. Insufficient vascular perfusion presents hypovolemia, hypoxia, hypotension, and impaired circulatory oxygen transport.
2. The normative cerebral perfusion pressure is 60–100 mm Hg. Impaired cerebral perfusion can cause weakness, altered mental status, restlessness, confusion, lethargy, impaired speech, decreased consciousness and a lower Glasgow Coma Scale score, decreased pupil reaction to light, seizures, difficulty swallowing (dysphagia), behavioral changes, and paralysis.
3. Impaired renal system perfusion can cause increased BUN, oliguria, anuria, blood pressure fluctuations, raised BUN/Creatinine ratio, and hematuria.
4. Poor heart and cardiac tissue perfusion can cause angina, abnormal arterial blood gasses, hypotension, tachycardia, tachypnea, and a sense of impending doom.
5. Poor gastrointestinal perfusion can cause nausea, diminished motility, absent bowel sounds, abdominal distention, and abdominal pain.
6. Intermittent claudication, weak or absent peripheral pulses, aches, pain, coolness, and numbness of the extremities, clammy and mottled skin, different blood pressure on both limbs, edema, and slow capillary refill times are symptoms of peripheral vascular system hypoperfusion (Burke, 2023).

Cerebral, cardiac, and peripheral hemostasis result from vascular constriction and spasm, blood clotting, and platelet plugs, stopping bleeding from wounds. Hemostasis is altered in hemolysis, elevated liver enzymes, low platelet count (HELLP) syndrome, congenital clotting disorders, increased blood viscosity, and platelet abnormalities. The postoperative period and immobility often impair the coagulation process/hemostasis. Treatment goals are to rectify and treat any curable causes and improve tissue perfusion.

Lead Selection for Cardiac Monitoring

The three-lead system, displaying lead I, II, III, or MCL1/MCL6, is conventional and most straightforward. Most ICU monitors use a five-electrode cable. The right lower limb electrode is the ground electrode on the torso, which has four electrodes. A chest lead position, generally V1, uses a fifth electrode for arrhythmia monitoring and helps diagnose pacemaker rhythms, broad QRS complex tachycardias, and bundle branch blocks (Cardiac Monitor Set-up and Lead-Placement, 2023).

The bedside EASI 12-lead consists of:

1. The E (brown) electrode on the lower part of the sternum in the fifth intercostal space (ICS).
2. The A (red) electrode on the left midaxillary line in the fifth ICS.
3. The S (black) electrode on the upper part of the sternum.
4. The I (white) electrode on the right midaxillary line in the fifth ICS.
5. The fifth (ground) electrode anywhere on the chest.

It continuously monitors all 12 heart views with five electrodes. Nevertheless, experts differ on replacing 12-lead ECGs, the gold standard of cardiac monitoring, with EASI-derived ones.

Vasoactive Medications Titration

1. Titration is raising or lowering a vasoactive drug infusion for a therapy.
2. Vasopressor is a drug class that causes arteriole vasoconstriction and raises BP.
3. Inotropes increase (positive) or decrease (negative) myocardial contractility. Negative inotropes like beta blockers decrease cardiac workload and BP, and positive inotropes like dopamine, dobutamine, epinephrine, and norepinephrine increase them.
4. Chronotrope affects the HR. Dobutamine is a positive chronotrope; Lopressor is negative.
5. Catecholamines are aromatic amines with sympathomimetic action like epinephrine, norepinephrine, dopamine, and dobutamine.
6. Adrenergics secrete epinephrine or norepinephrine.

SBP drops of > 30mm Hg or MAP drops of 60–65mm Hg can cause end-organ failure, necessitating vasoactive medications. Vasoactive drugs treat hypertensive crises, flash pulmonary edema, sepsis, shock states, atrial fibrillation with rapid ventricular response, supraventricular tachycardia, heart failure, and hemodynamic instability.

Treat hypovolemia and volume loss before taking a vasopressor. If fluid status is unknown, evaluate vasoactive drip efficacy hemodynamically. Patients require continuous monitoring of heart, BP, and oxygen saturation. Emergency resuscitation tools and medicines are essential for managing drug reactions.

Dopamine is an intrinsically produced precursor of norepinephrine. When shock is due to unknown causes and used for central hypotension, heart failure, and renal and mesenteric perfusion, dopamine is a good first-line drug of choice. In higher doses, it acts more like an alpha agonist; in low doses, it works like a beta agonist.

Dopamine titration: 400 mg is mixed in 250 mL/D5W, making 1600 mcg/ml. Action begins at 5 minutes, half-life is 2 minutes. The dosage is 2-20 mcg/kg/min, typically starting at 5 mcg/kg/min. Check urine output hourly.

Dobutamine is a first-line inotropic adrenergic agonist. Dobutamine treats cardiogenic shock and hypotension. A BP fall (hypotension) can happen with hypovolemia (low fluid volume). If hypotension occurs, stop the infusion and manage fluid volume losses. The medication can cause tachycardia and headache. Those allergic to sulfite should avoid it. Its half-life is 2 minutes, and the onset is 1–2 minutes. Mix 500 mg in 250 ml D5W for a 2000 mcg/ml infusion. Start the drip at 1–2 mcg/kg/min and titrate to 40 mcg/kg/min.

Nitroglycerin, a nitrate, dilates coronary arteries and lowers preload. It is an anti-anginal, antihypertensive, and vasodilator. It is the drug of choice for cocaine-induced MI. Always prepare the infusion in a glass bottle with vented tubing. It is available as a premixed 50 mg/250 ml D5W (200 mcg/ml). The beginning dose is 10–20 mcg/min or 3-6 ml/hr. Use cautiously with oral nitrates, inferior wall MI, and sexual performance-enhancing medications to avoid life-threatening hypotension.

QTc Intervals

The QT interval includes the ventricular electrical events such as the QRS complex, the ST segment, and the T wave. Its duration is proportionate to the HR. The faster the heart rate, the shorter the QT interval. Conversely, the QT interval is long when the heart rate is slow. The QT interval generally comprises about 40% of each cardiac cycle (the R-R interval).

As the QT interval varies with the heart rate, a corrected QT interval, or QTc, assesses for absolute QT prolongation.

To account for heart rate variances, divide the QT interval by the square root of the R-R interval (in seconds). The algorithm works best between 50 and 120 beats/minute; it is less precise at higher heart rates.

The typical value for the QTc in men is ≤ 0.44 seconds and ≤ 0.45 to 0.46 seconds in women. Any medication that can prolong the QT interval must not exceed it by more than 500 milliseconds during therapy (550 milliseconds with an underlying bundle branch block) to reduce the possibility of ventricular dysrhythmias.

Patients with prolonged QT intervals may have a unique form of ventricular tachycardia (VT), Torsade de pointes, initiated by a premature ventricular contraction that falls during the elongated T wave. Some drugs that prolong QT interval include:

1. Tricyclic antidepressants
2. Erythromycin, quinolone antibiotics
3. Antihistamines with these antibiotics
4. Sotalol
5. Quinidine
6. Procainamide

ST Segment

The STsegment begins from the J point ((meeting point of the QRS complex and ST segment) to the beginning of the T wave. It corresponds to the plateau phase of an action potential. ST-segment elevation means J-point elevation of > 1 mm in limb leads and > 2 mm in V1-V3. Causes are:

1. Myocardial infarction
2. Prinzmetal angina (coronary vasospasm)
3. Tako-tsubo cardiomyopathy
4. Pericarditis
5. Left bundle branch block
6. Left ventricular hypertrophy

ST-segment depression is depression of the J point of > 1mm. Some of the causes are:

1. Exercise
2. Acute ischemia with upsloping ST depression and prominent T wave (de Winter's sign)
3. NSTEMI
4. STEMI as a reciprocal to ST elevation
5. Hypokalaemia and raised sympathetic tone
6. Digoxin
7. Left ventricular hypertrophy

Dysrhythmias

Atrial arrhythmias occur when the sinoatrial node, the heart's natural pacemaker, doesn't produce enough impulses. Atrial arrhythmias include flutter, fibrillation, supraventricular tachycardia, and premature atrial contractions (PAC).

Atrial Flutter

ECG

Atrial flutter shows abnormal P waves, sawtooth-like flutter waves, unmeasurable PR interval, and uniform QRS complexes 0.06–0.12 seconds long. The rhythm is regular.

Causes

1. Aging
2. COPD
3. Mitral valve defect
4. Cardiomyopathy
5. Ischemia

Symptoms

1. Weakness
2. Anxiety
3. Dyspnea
4. Palpitations
5. Angina
6. Syncope

Complications

1. Atrial clots
2. Pulmonary embolisms
3. Cerebrovascular accident
4. Cardiac output drops

Management

1. Anticoagulant therapy
2. Cardioversion
3. Antiarrhythmic drugs, beta blockers/digitalis

Atrial Fibrillation

ECG

The rhythm is irregular; nonexistent P waves are replaced with f waves, there is an absent PR interval, and uniform QRS complexes are 0.06 to 0.12 seconds long.

Causes

1. Hypertension
2. Heart failure
3. Impaired sinus node functioning
4. Hypoxia
5. Mitral valve defect
6. Pericarditis
7. Rheumatic heart disease
8. Coronary artery disease
9. Hyperthyroidism
10. Aging
11. Pulmonary embolism

Symptoms

1. Chest tightness
2. Palpitations
3. Dyspnea
4. Fluttering in the chest
5. Dizziness
6. Confusion
7. Syncope

Complications

Complications are the same as atrial flutter.

Management

1. Beta blockers, calcium channel blockers, or digoxin to control HR
2. Intravenous verapamil for rapid reduction in HR
3. Cardioversion
4. Supplemental oxygen
5. Antithrombotic medications

Premature atrial contractions (PAC)

ECG

PAC happens when the p wave occurs prematurely. After this premature p wave, there is a compensatory pause.

The cardiac rate is typically normal, but the cardiac rhythm is irregular because of the compensatory pause. The p wave occurs prior to each QRS complex, and it is typically upright but not always with its normal shape. The PR interval is from 0.12 to 0.20 seconds. The QRS complexes look alike, and their length ranges from 0.06 to 0.12 seconds.

Quiz

1. Which is an indication for alpha-adrenergic blockers?

   A. Decreased stroke volume
   B. Increased cardiac afterload
   C. Diminished cardiac afterload
   D. Increased cardiac preload

2. Which cardiac cycle can you listen to the murmur of mitral insufficiency?

   A. During diastole
   B. During systole
   C. Throughout the cardiac cycle
   D. None of these

3. Which type of dysrhythmia is common in mitral insufficiency?

    A. AV block II degree
    B. Complete heart block
    C. AV dissociation
    D. AFib

4. Which can treat coronary vasospasm caused by variant (prinzmetal's) angina?

    A. Calcium-channel blockers (CCBs)
    B. Alpha blockers
    C. Beta blockers
    D. Cholinergic agents

5. If the ECG shows ST segment elevation in leads II, III, and aVF, which wall of the heart is the patient experiencing an infarction?

    A. Anterior
    B. Inferior
    C. Posterior
    D. Lateral

Answers

1. C. Alpha-adrenergic blockers ameliorate reduce cardiac afterload in hypertensive crisis. You may use the assessment approach to answer this question. As the name suggests, alpha-adrenergic blockers block alpha-adrenergic receptors that contract vascular wall muscles, causing vasodilation. In conditions with diminished cardiac afterload, such as hypertensive crisis, less blood is pumped into the circulation, causing cerebral hypoperfusion. Alpha blockers can dilate vessels and improve circulation.
2. B. Mitral insufficiency causes a systolic murmur.
3. D. An irregular AFib can occur with mitral insufficiency.
4. A. CCBs can treat the vasospasm caused by variant angina.
5. B. The patient has an inferior wall infarction.

Chapter Three:
Pulmonary System

Acute Respiratory Distress Syndrome (ARDS)

Acute respiratory distress syndrome (ARDS) is an acute, life-threatening condition characterized by poor oxygenation and bilateral lung infiltrates. Microscopy reveals capillary endothelial and diffuse alveolar (lung cell) damage, which leads to increased alveolar-capillary leakage, interstitial edema, and reduced lung compliance in the absence of primary cardiogenic causes of lung edema.

In ARDS, oxygen in arterial blood (PaO2) to the fraction of the oxygen in the inspired air (FiO2) or PaO2/FiO2 ratio is < 200 mm Hg. Patients may eventually develop pulmonary hypertension, reduced right ventricular compliance and cardiac output, and increased mortality.

Causes

1. *Lung infection or aspiration*
2. Events triggering systemic inflammation

   a. Sepsis
   b. Trauma
   c. Large transfusion

    d. Drowning
    e. Drug overdose
    f. Fat embolism
    g. Inhalation of toxic fumes
        h. Pancreatitis

Risk Factors

1. Age
2. Female gender
3. Smoking
4. Alcohol

The ARDS incidence in the US ranges from 64.2–78.9 cases/100,000 person-years (Diamond et al., 2024). Around 75% of cases are moderate/severe. Gross pooled mortality rate for all the studies is 43% (Wang et al., 2021).

Symptoms

Dyspnea and progressively deteriorating hypoxia (within hours to days), often needing mechanical ventilation and ICU care.

1. Increased effort of breathing
2. Signs
3. Persisting hypoxia despite 100% oxygen
4. Central or peripheral cyanosis
5. Tachycardia
6. Altered mental status
7. Bibasilar/diffuse rales on chest auscultation

Diagnosis

1. Acute onset
2. Bilateral lung infiltrates on chest X-ray of non-cardiac origin
3. PaO/FiO ratio < 300 mm Hg

a. mild (PaO2/FiO2: 200–300 mm Hg)
b. Moderate (PaO2/FiO2: 100–200 mm Hg)
c. Severe (PaO2/FiO2 < 100 mm Hg

4. A chest CT scan revealing pneumothorax/pleural effusions/mediastinal lymphadenopathy/barotrauma can pinpoint the pulmonary origin of infiltrates.
5. Non-invasive (better) cardiac echocardiography, thoracic bioimpedance, or pulse contour analysis to exclude CHF/find its contributory effects in the process.
6. Bronchoscopy to assess pulmonary infections and obtain culture material.
7. Other laboratory and radiographic tests consider:

a. The underlying cause, if identifiable
b. Associated multi-organ failure, such as renal, hepatic, and failure of blood cell productions

Nursing Care Plan

Diagnosis

8. Disabled gas exchange due to ineffective breathing
1. Ineffective airway clearance
2. Aspiration
3. Reduced activity tolerance
4. Anxiety (mild, moderate, severe, panic)

Interventions

1. Nutritional support
2. Ventilation maintenance
3. Barotrauma monitoring
4. Oral cavity suction
5. Antibiotics administration
6. Prevention of

    a. DVT

    b. Stress ulcer

    c. Aspiration

    d. Pneumonia

7. Blood chemistry and fluid monitoring

Seek Help

1. Hypotension
2. Persistent hypoxia
3. Raised peak airway pressures
4. Reduced urine output
5. High temperature
6. Unresponsive patient

Prognosis

Most patients have guarded outcomes. Those who recover have a prolonged recovery, with significant weakness, wasting, and nerve damage. Personnel involved:

1. Dietitian and nutritionist
2. Respiratory therapist
3. Pharmacist
4. Pulmonologist
5. Nephrologist
6. Nurses (to monitor and move the patient and educate the family)
7. Physical therapist
8. Tracheostomy nurse (to help maintain tracheostomy and weaning).
9. Mental health nurse (to assess depression/anxiety/other psychosocial issues).

Asthma

Asthma is a common childhood disease associated with atopy, such as eczema and hay fever. It ranges from a mild, occasional wheeze to an acute, life-threatening airway closure.

Causes

1. Genetic predisposition
2. Personal/close family history of atopy (allergies such as eczema, hay fever, and asthma)
3. Smoking and air pollution

The transition from pediatric asthma to asthma in adulthood is complex and ill-understood. A multifactorial pathology involving genetics and environmental exposure is suggested.

Risk Factors

Approximately 40% of children suffer from wheezing. Asthma is wheezing reversible by beta-2 agonists is termed asthma, regardless of the lung function tests.

Diagnosis

1. Assess asthma severity/deterioration with pulse oximetry. Mechanical lag/physiological lung reserve can delay pulse oximetry pO2 drops. Not knowing this can delay treatment and cause respiratory failure.
2. Compare peak flow measures to a nomogram and normal baseline functions.
3. Check urea and electrolytes for high-dose/repeat salbutamol. Salbutamol induces transient hypokalemia.
4. Check chest X-ray to rule out foreign bodies and infections as causes of wheezing.

Spirometry is best for diagnosing an obstructive pattern that salbutamol partially or totally resolves.

Management

1. Calm the patient; quieten the surroundings.
2. Eliminate potential allergen sources (allergy testing).
3. Bronchodilators like beta-2 agonists and muscarinic antagonists (salbutamol and ipratropium bromide)
4. Anti-inflammatories like inhaled steroids (beclometasone)
5. Weight loss
6. Stop smoking
7. Occupational modifications
8. Asthma self-monitoring

Nursing Care Plan

Nursing care plan involves:

Assessment

1. History of a wheeze/cough aggravated by allergies (pollen), exercise, and cold.
2. A diurnal variation with worsening of nocturnal symptoms
3. During an acute exacerbation

    a. Mild tachycardia
    b. Varying degrees of respiratory distress
    c. Bilateral, expiratory wheeze on auscultation
    d. Silent chest in life-threatening asthma signifies an absence of air entry.

Diagnosis

1. Chest discomfort/tightness
2. Dyspnea and wheeze
3. Cough
4. Cyanosis
5. Tachypnea and tachycardia
6. Working of accessory respiratory muscles
7. Tripod position (sitting forward to open their airways)

Interventions

1. Monitor oxygen status
2. Auscultate lungs
3. Assess respiratory distress
4. Position the patient upright
5. Administer prescribed medications

Seek Help

1. Respiratory distress
2. Silent chest on auscultation
3. Low oxygen saturation
4. Cyanosis

Desired Outcome

1. Normal breathing
2. Normal oxygen saturation
3. No wheeze
4. No breathing distress

Evaluation

Admit the patient if they need nebulized salbutamol and are not on it. Monitor severe or life-threatening asthmatics to prevent relapse once the medication wears off.

1. Auscultate wheeze
2. Medication adherence
3. Temperature
4. Vitals
5. Oxygen saturation
6. ABG

Nursing Management Errors

1. Not assessing the inhaler technique
2. Forgetting to remove the nebulizer mask after use
3. Neglecting to emphasize maintenance therapy with inhaled steroids even when the patient is well

Prognosis

Well-managed asthma is a reversible disorder.

1. School and work days absenteeism
2. Increasing healthcare costs
3. Debilitating chronic airway problem due to poor lifestyle and management
4. Mortality is one out of every 100,000 persons. It is due to

   a. Poor lung function
   b. Poor management
   c. Medication non-compliance
   d. Smoking
   e. Drug abuse

Evidence-Based Medicine

1. Patient compliance with medications is a significant problem. *Patient education is critical to success* (Hashmi et al., 2023). Nurses and pharmacists can impart training on monitoring, inhaler use, home nebulizer techniques, and environmental modifications. They can also distribute patient education materials. Nurses can help improve self-confidence, knowledge, and behavioral adjustments.
2. Reduce asthma attacks by controlling the environment and avoiding triggers.

COPD Exacerbation

The Global Initiative for COPD considers it a manageable and curable condition with some major extrapulmonary effects that can add to the disease's severity.

COPD can be chronic bronchitis and emphysema. However, many have overlapping signs and symptoms.

Chronic Bronchitis (Blue Bloaters)

Pollutants or allergens stimulate sputum production by the mucus-secreting glands and goblet cells.

1. Cough and sputum production for at least three months in each of two consecutive years.
2. Viral, bacterial, and mycoplasmal infections precipitate acute exacerbations of chronic bronchitis.

Emphysema (Pink Puffers)

Emphysema is an abnormal enlargement of airways beyond the terminal bronchioles with alveolar wall damage. Patients become increasingly breathless.

Causes

1. Smoking
2. Occupational exposure and air pollution
3. Genetic deficiency of alpha1-antitrypsin (it protects the lung from injury)

Symptoms

1. Variably progressive disease with

   a. *Chronic cough: the hallmark of COPD*
   b. Sputum production
   c. Exertional dyspnea progresses to dyspnea at rest
   d. Weight loss

Diagnosis

1. Health history
2. Pulmonary function studies
3. Spirometry: forced expiratory volume over 1 second (FEV1)/forced vital capacity (FVC)
4. ABG
5. Chest X-ray
6. Screening for alpha1-antitrypsin deficiency in < 45 years for those with a strong COPD family history.
7. ECG: features of right ventricular hypertrophy and P-pulmonale (P waves ≥ 2.5 mm in leads II, III, and aVF).

Management of Exacerbations

1. First-line therapy: adjusting bronchodilator medications.
2. Hospitalization under the following conditions

   a. Acute exacerbation with severe dyspnea not responding to therapy

     b. Confusion/lethargy
     c. Overworking of respiratory muscle
     d. Paradoxical chest wall movement
     e. Peripheral edema

3. Supplemental oxygen therapy
4. Antibiotics in increased dyspnea, sputum production, and sputum purulence

Nursing Care Plan

Nursing management involves the following.

Priorities

1. Airway patency
2. Improved nutritional intake
3. Prevention of complications and progression
4. Information is provided about the disease process/prognosis and treatment regimen

Assessment

Rapid and accurate assessments include:

1. Risk factors
2. Medical history past and present
3. Symptoms and signs of COPD and their severity
4. Patients' knowledge of the disease
5. Vitals
6. Breath sounds and patterns.

Diagnosis

1. Diagnosis involves

   a. Impaired gas exchange
   b. Ineffective airway clearance
   c. Ineffective breathing pattern
   d. Lack of self-care
   e. Activity intolerance

Interventions

1. Patient and family education
2. Airway patency

   a. Administer bronchodilators and corticosteroids properly; consider potential side effects.
   b. Direct or controlled coughing instructions, which reduces fatigue
   c. Breathing pattern improvement:
   d. Inspiratory muscle training
   e. Diaphragmatic breathing reduces respiratory rate, improves alveolar ventilation, and may expel air during expiration
   f. Pursed lip breathing controls the rate and depth of respiration

3. Activity tolerance

   a. Pace daily activities with periodic rest; use support devices to reduce energy expenditure
   b. Exercise training to strengthen muscles and improve exercise tolerance and endurance
   c. Walking aids

4. Potential complications avoidance

   a. Observe cognitive changes
   b. Monitor pulse oximetry values

c. Prevent infection, including immunization against influenza and pneumonia

Desired Outcome

1. Optimization in gas exchange
2. Clearing the airway
3. Improved breathing
4. Self-care competence
5. Reduced activity intolerance
6. Proper ventilation/oxygen for self-care
7. Adequate nutrition
8. Treat/prevent infection
9. Grasp of disease, prognosis, and treatment
10. Plan for post-discharge requirements:

    a. Risks of smoking acknowledged
    b. Find and enroll in smoking cessation resources
    c. Minimize/abolish exposures
    d. States need for fluids
    e. Infection-free
    f. Breathing technique practice; functioning with reduced breathing difficulties

Documentation

1. Assessment and laboratory findings
2. Conditions restricting oxygen supply
3. Care plan, modifications, and specific interventions
4. Amount of supplemental oxygen
5. Treatment and teaching responses
6. Teaching plan
7. Outcome achievement/progress

Minimally-Invasive Thoracic Surgery

Grossly invasive thoracotomy is now replaced with minimally invasive video-assisted thoracoscopic surgery (VATS). It has improved patient experiences and outcomes worldwide. However, a non-intubated VATS requires careful planning, nursing, and team cooperation.

Role of Circulating Nurses

1. Review the ward's medical records.
2. Get the surgery plan.
3. Work with patients
4. Visit before surgery.
5. Introduce themselves.
6. Check patients' emotional and physical well-being a day before surgery.
7. Discuss the technique, doctors, and benefits of non-intubated anesthesia.
8. Include the operating room, operative posture, etc., in the discussion.
9. Share additional success stories with the patient to relax them and promote confidence.
10. Tell patients that non-intubated anesthetic lets them wake up for surgery, lowering anxiety.

Role of Equipment Nurse

A lobectomy involves two or three ports. The observation port, operational port, and auxiliary port create an isosceles triangle between the 6th–7th, 4th–5th, and 6th–7th intercostal cartilages. A 30° thoracoscope views the thoracic cavity.

1. Gives the surgeon a lubricated incision protection sleeve for each port
2. Gives the surgeon a gauze pad with a toothed oval clamp retaining 1/4 of it to press the lung tissue to expose the surgical site after an incision is made
3. Gives the surgeon an endoscopic needle with a 1% Lidocaine syringe (3-5mL) to block the vagus nerve. Both the nurse and the surgeon must monitor medicine concentration and dosage
4. Hands the endoscopic siphon head to the assistant to facilitate the exposure

5. Installs the Johnson & Johnson pleural automatic cutter & stapler before passing it to the operator
6. Hands an ultrasonic scalpel to the operator during the lower lobe resection to separate the inferior pulmonary ligament, slowly exposing the inferior pulmonary vein
7. Hands thoracoscopic forceps to the operator to complete the vascular exploration
8. Passes the surgeon a pleural automatic cutter and stapler to the surgeon to separate the inferior pulmonary artery and vein and the lower lobe bronchus
9. Hands the different vessel-separating clamps to the operator, tallying with the operation steps during the resection of other lung lobes
10. Helps select different types of cartridges during lobe resection based on tissue thickness
11. Hands the endosurgical extraction bag after lobectomy to collect body tissues
12. Helps prepare chest tubes and chest drainage bottles
13. Counts equipment, blood pads, and gauze routinely. The incision is closed when the count tallies
14. Cleans and maintains equipment and instruments

Obstructive Sleep Apnea

A blocked upper airway during sleep causes *obstructive sleep apnea (OSA)*, the most prevalent kind. *Central sleep apnea (CSA)* occurs when the brain and breathing muscles briefly disconnect.

Symptoms

1. Sleep-related breathing ceases or resumes (usually seen by another)
2. Gasping during sleep
3. Loud snoring
4. Morning dry mouth
5. Daytime fatigue and drowsiness
6. Sleep deprivation

Risk Factors

1. Constricted air passages/tonsillar enlargement
2. Wide/thick-necked persons
3. Male
4. Aging
5. Obesity
6. Smoking
7. Asthma, HTN, CHF

Diagnosis

1. Sleep study
2. Medical history
3. Physical examination

Management

1. Mild cases

   a. Lifestyle modifications
   b. Losing weight
   c. Treating nasal allergies
   d. Smoking cessation

2. Moderate to severe sleep apnea

   a. Continuous positive airway pressure (CPAP)
   b. Airway pressure devices
   c. Supplemental oxygen
   d. Using an oral device

Nursing Care Plan

Diagnosis

Ineffective Breathing

The obstructed airways collapse during sleep, ensuing ineffective breathing and lowering oxygenation. Body position can also affect lung expansion.

Evidence

1. Reduced RR
2. Cyanosis
3. Sleep apnea
4. Hypoventilation
5. Hypoxia

Assessment

1. Assess frequency and pattern of breathing to understand disease progression. Mild sleep apnea is 5–10 apnea events/hour.
2. Assess diagnostic tests like night-time polysomnography and home sleep tests.

Interventions

1. Encourage sleeping in a side-lying position instead of supine with forward/backward neck bending.
2. Appraise easier-to-use oral devices to keep the throat open and bring the jaw forward, relieving obstruction.
3. Check oxygen saturation during sleep with an apnea monitor and pulse oximeter.
4. Administer prescribed medications like methylxanthine (relaxes smooth muscles).

Desired Outcome

1. The patient will perform interventions to check sleep apnea.
2. The patient will maintain an effective breathing pattern, rhythm, and rate.

Impaired Gas Exchange

Evidence

1. Hypoxia
2. Reduced oxygen saturation
3. Cyanosis
4. Altered arterial pH
5. Altered respiratory depth and rhythm

Assessment

1. Assess the patient's respiratory and other parameters like vital signs, ABGs, and SpO2.
2. Assess experiences related to poor sleep, such as daytime sleepiness, tiredness, difficulty focusing, and hampered sleep patterns related to OSA.

Interventions

1. Avoid bedtime sedatives to avoid respiratory depression.
2. Use the CPAP machine following directions. It adjusts the pressure to help maintain airflow during sleep.
3. Consider surgical options as a last resort, including implants, tissue removal, jaw repositioning, or tracheostomy.
4. Administer supplemental oxygen as recommended.

Desired Outcome

1. Patients will have reduced apneic episodes while sleeping.
2. Patients will show normal SpO2 during sleep.

Knowledge Deficiency

Evidence

1. Inaccurate use of CPAP/BiPAP
2. Inaccurate execution of instructions
3. Inaccurate remarks about sleep apnea
4. Lifestyle recommendation non-compliance

Assessment

1. Assess the patient's knowledge about OSA to determine any necessary additional information and correct misinformation.
2. Assess the patient's commitment to wearing the recommended device and execute lifestyle modifications. Family support is paramount.

Interventions

1. Educate about maintaining sleep/wake times, keeping the environment quiet, cool, and dark, reducing caffeine intake in the evening, and eating early.
2. Manage chronic conditions like asthma, diabetes, CHF, and hypertension.
3. Motivate necessary lifestyle changes.
4. Provide resources for free/low-cost supplies.

Desired Outcome

1. The patient will state their risk factors concerning sleep apnea.
2. The patient will use their CPAP machine correctly.

Pleural Space Complications

Hemothorax

Hemothorax refers to blood in the pleural space.

Causes

1. Blunt/penetrating trauma
2. Disease
3. Iatrogenic
4. Spontaneous

Pneumothorax

In pneumothorax, the pleural space is exposed to positive atmospheric pressure following a breach in the parietal/visceral pleura. The lung or a portion of it collapses due to a loss of negative pleural pressure. In tension pneumothorax, a lacerated lung or minor chest wall opening or wound draws air into the pleural area.

Causes

1. Blunt chest wall trauma
2. COPD
3. Astma
4. Cystic fibrosis

Empyema

In Empyema, pus collects in the pleural cavity. It is usually associated with pneumonia but can also develop after thoracic surgery or trauma.

Causes

1. Bacterial pneumonia
2. Lung abscess
3. Chest surgery/injuries getting infected

Chylothorax

Chylothorax is a rare and serious condition of lymph (chyle) accumulating in the chest cavity.

Causes

1. Lymphatic disorders/malformations
2. Genetic causes
3. Lymphoma

Nursing Care Plan

Risk Factor Awareness

1. Musculoskeletal injury
2. Chest drainage system/malfunction
3. Absent safety education/precautions
4. Thoracotomy

Priorities

1. Proper ventilation and airway patency
2. Effective pain assessment and management
3. Care for wounds and check for infection
4. Preventing and tracking complications
5. Explain the disease and therapy

Assessment

1. Hemothorax

    a. Breathing shortness/difficulty
    b. Stabbing chest pain/chest heaviness
    c. Diminished breath sounds on the affected side
    d. Dullness to percussion both front and back laterally (fluid)

    e. Lowered oxygen saturation

    f. Shock

        i. Hypotension

        ii. Tachycardia

        iii. Rapid, weak pulse

        iv. Pale/clammy skin

2. Pneumothorax

    a. Sharply acute chest pain

    b. Breathlessness

    c. Decreased/absent breath sounds

    d. Hyperresonant on percussion (air)

    e. Asymmetrical chest motion

    f. Cyanosis, abnormal ABGs

3. Jugular vein distention (tension pneumothorax)

Diagnosis

Nursing diagnosis is based on clinical judgment and understanding of the uniqueness of health conditions. The nurse's clinical expertise and inferences shape the care plan and set priorities.

Interventions

Improve Breathing Pattern

Determining the cause, such as spontaneous collapse, trauma, malignancy, infection, or mechanical ventilation complications, is necessary for choosing appropriate therapeutic measures.

1. Assess respiratory function and vital signs.
2. Maintain a synchronous respiratory pattern for mechanical ventilators. Notice airway pressure changes.

3. Assess breath sounds, chest motions, and tracheal position. In a supine patient, lower yourself to be at level with the client.
4. Assess for fremitus (vibration), which are reduced in fluid-filled or consolidated tissue.
5. Assess mental and cardiac status frequently. Changes in a mental status may indicate respiratory distress in malfunctioning chest drainage system.
6. Perform splinting painful areas to assuage pain during coughing and deep breathing.
7. Keep the head of the bed elevated. Turn the client to the affected side. Encourage them to sit up as much as possible.
8. Maintain calmness; help the client assume control by breathing slowly to address the physiological effects of hypoxia, expressed as anxiety or fear (Vera, 2023).
9. Administer humidified oxygen if indicated.
10. Provide a low-carbohydrate, high-fat diet, if recommended.
11. Administer pain medications per order.

Manage Patients with Chest Tube

1. Urgent cases need immediate needle decompression. Chest tube drainage and suction expand the lung and remove air or fluid.
2. Note whether a dry seal/water seal system is used.
3. Check the suction control chamber for the precise suction amount. Monitor fluid level in the water-seal chamber and keep it at the prescribed level.
4. Dial dry suction levels as prescribed. Note if the water-seal chamber is bubbling during expiration (the desired action). Bubbling decreases with lung expansion.
5. Identify the location of the air leak by clamping the catheter distal to exit from the chest.
6. Place petrolatum gauze around the insertion as ordered.
7. Clamp the catheter in a stepwise manner down toward the drainage unit for persistent air leak.
8. Seal connection sites securely with lengthwise tape or bands per policy.
9. Monitor the tidaling of the water-seal chamber.

10. Ensure the tubing is not kinked or hanging below the entrance to the drainage container.
11. Assess the drainage and the need for milking.
12. Strip tubes carefully per protocol, minimizing excess negative pressure.
13. Place a sterile occlusive dressing on the insertion site after drainage removal.
14. Observe signs and symptoms of recurrence.
15. Refer/assist in pulmonary rehabilitation, as recommended.

Desired Outcome

1. The client will establish a normal/effective breathing rhythm with normal ABGs.
2. The client will not have cyanosis/hypoxia symptoms.
3. The client's chest x-ray will show lung expansion.
4. The client will have good gas exchange and ventilatory function, shown by normal RRs, mental clarity, and orientation.

Pulmonary Embolism

Pulmonary embolism (PE) occurs when a thrombus (embolus) in the venous system or on the right side of the heart obstructs the flow of blood to the pulmonary artery or one of its branches. The emboli can be fat, air, septic, or amniotic fluid (pregnancy).

Causes

1. Trauma
2. Procedures such as orthopedic, major abdominal, pelvic, and gynecologic surgeries
3. Hypercoagulable states
4. Extended immobility

Symptoms

1. Dyspnea
2. Sudden chest pain (pleuritic)
3. Tachycardia
4. Tachypnea

Preventative Treatment

1. Avoiding venous stasis with active leg exercises/early mobilization
2. Using sequential compression devices
3. Adopting mechanical prophylaxis static or dynamic
4. Using graduated compression stockings
5. Administering anticoagulant

Nursing Care Plan

Assessment

All in-hospital patients must be assessed for risk factors for PE/DVT.

1. History of cardiovascular disease in the family/patient
2. Medications that increase the risk
3. Warmth, redness, and inflammation in extremities.

Diagnosis

1. Ineffective peripheral tissue perfusion
2. Risk for shock
3. Acute pleuritic pain

Interventions

1. Encourage active and passive leg exercises to check venous stasis.
2. Monitor thrombolytic and anticoagulant therapy through INR or PTT.
3. Reposition the patient frequently to improve the ventilation-perfusion ratio.
4. Assess pulse oximetry values and hypoxic signs.
5. Urge the patient to discuss relevant concerns/anxiety.

Desired Outcome

1. Improve perfusion
2. State comprehension of condition, therapy mode, and drug side effects
3. Show hemodynamic stability
4. Report pain is alleviated/controlled
5. Maintain prescribed pharmacologic advice

Discharge Education

1. Check recurrences by early reporting signs and symptoms.
2. Check adherence to the prescribed management plan.
3. Monitor residual PE effects and recovery.
4. Remind the patient about the need for PE follow-up appointments.

Pulmonary Hypertension

The Sixth World Symposium on Pulmonary Hypertension (WSPH) defines pulmonary hypertension (PAH) as mean pulmonary arterial pressure (mPAP) > 20 mm Hg (Kovacs and Olschewski, 2021).

Types

1. Idiopathic (IPAH) accounts for 30%–50% of PAH cases.

2. Heritable PAH (HPAH) is confirmed if two/more family members are diagnosed with PAH.
3. Some drugs and toxins can induce PAH.
4. PAH is associated with other diseases (connective tissue disease, HIV, congenital heart disease, portal hypertension, etc.).

Stiff and thickened pulmonary artery walls raise *pulmonary vascular resistance (PVR), the hallmark of PAH*. Subsequent RV hypertrophy (RVH) reduces forward blood flow, CO, tricuspid regurgitation (TR), and right heart failure (RHF).

Symptoms

1. Subtle symptoms are present for years before overt manifestations. Unexplained dyspnea is often mistaken for asthma.
2. Weakness
3. Exercise intolerance
4. Lightheadedness
5. Syncope
6. Tachypnea
7. Anxiety

Signs

1. The first sign is a loud pulmonic component of the second heart sound (P2), best heard at the right second intercostal space.
2. A holosystolic murmur (TR) at the lower left sternal border/apex (RVH)
3. Features of RHF
4. Cyanosis and cool extremities (Diminished CO)

The nursing care of patients corresponds with the World Health Organization (WHO) Group 1 form of PH (there are five) called PAH.

Diagnosis

The ECG may show signs of right ventricular hypertrophy or strain. A 2D echocardiography with Doppler flow studies can detect tricuspid regurgitation, pulmonary artery pressure, RV dilation, and RV hypertrophy, making it an essential PAH screening tool. However, cardiac catheterization is the gold standard for PAH diagnosis.

A sleep apnea study is recommended, as nocturnal hypoxia and sleep apnea are found in 70–80% of patients with PAH. A ventilation-perfusion (V/Q) imaging scan rules out chronic thromboembolic PAH (O'Leary, 2021).

Nursing Care Plan

Interventions

Prevent Falls

Falls due to syncopal episodes, shortness of breath, and deconditioning increase risks of trauma.

1. Monitor patients' BP frequently; commence fall prevention measures.
2. Instruct the patient to call for assistance before getting out of bed.
3. Avoid temperature extremes such as hot showers and saunas, which may cause hypotension and syncope due to vasodilation.
4. Encourage physical activity in stable patients with optimal medication.

Prevent Infection

Assess and maintain catheter sterility and proper hand hygiene, and monitor catheter insertion sites for infection.

Evaluation

IV epoprostenol and prostacyclin require continuous evaluation, management, and notification of PAH signs and symptoms, adverse reactions, BP, heart rate, heart rhythm, and oxygen saturation levels. Abrupt Epoprostenol cessation can rebound PAH.

1. Check daily weights, intake, and output every shift, and serum electrolytes.
2. Continuous telemetry may be needed to monitor atrial dysrhythmias.

Education

Patient and caregiver education is an integral nursing component.

1. Advise healthy diet, smoking cessation, and vaccination against influenza and pneumococcal pneumonia.
2. Alert against high altitudes/air travel due to hypoxemia.
3. Instruct to avoid over-the-counter medications (decongestants or herbal remedies such as Ephedra, dong quai, St. John's wort, and ginseng)
4. Monitor for anxiety and depression and coping strategies.

Respiratory Depression

The *nursing care plan* for acute respiratory failure is essential to managing the challenging and potentially fatal condition. To start the care plan, include a comprehensive nursing assessment comprising respiratory history, physical examination, neurological and cardiac assessment, respiratory function tests, and psychosocial evaluation. This examination determines the causes and contributors of acute respiratory failure.

Assessment findings help formulate nursing diagnosis, including impaired gas exchange, ineffective airway clearance, anxiety, and infection risks. Diagnoses give a framework for planning and executing nursing interventions.

Improving oxygenation, ventilation, airway clearance, emotional support to lessen anxiety, and infection prevention are *nursing interventions*. These therapies may include supplementary oxygen, lung expansion positioning, coughing and deep breathing exercises, chest physiotherapy, medicines, and infection control.

Respiratory Failure

Acute respiratory failure, a life-threatening condition, occurs when the respiratory system cannot meet the patient's oxygenation, ventilation, or metabolic needs. Weaning failure involves failing a spontaneous breathing trial or needing reintubation within 48 hours of extubation. Chronic respiratory failure persists. It grows slowly and requires long-term care.

Hypoxemic respiratory failure is poor capillary-alveoli oxygen exchange. With a normal or low partial pressure of arterial carbon dioxide (PaCo2), PaO2 will be less than 60 mm Hg.

Hypercapnic respiratory failure causes acidosis by ventilatory failure with PaCO2 over 45 mm Hg.

Causes

1. Chest/lung/brain injury (choking, drowning, or being hit in the chest)
2. Drug/alcohol overdose
3. Toxic fume/smoke
4. Lung disease/infection(ARDS/COPD/cystic fibrosis/pneumonia)
5. Muscle and nerve damage (amyotrophic lateral sclerosis (ALS), spinal cord injuries, stroke, myasthenia gravis, etc.)
6. Scoliosis/other spine problems
7. Pulmonary embolism

Risks

1. Long-term respiratory problems like COPD/asthma
2. Smoking/vaping/e-cigarette/marijuana/scented candle fumes

3. Excessive drinking
4. A family history of respiratory problems
5. Compromised immune system
6. Recent surgical procedure

Symptoms

1. Cyanosis
2. Breathing shortness
3. Confusion
4. Irregular beats
5. Rapid/overly slow breathing
6. Tightness of chest
7. Drowsiness/syncope

Diagnosis

1. CBC
2. Pulse oximetry
3. ABG
4. Chest X-ray
5. ECG

Management of Acute Respiratory Failure

1. Assess the ABCs (airway, breathing, and circulation) to identify the priority.
2. A PaO2 of 60 mm Hg/an oxygen saturation (SaO2) of 90% is obtained with oxygen through

   a. Nasal cannula
   b. Simple face mask
   c. Non-rebreather mask
   d. High-flow nasal cannula

3. Avoid over-oxygenation.
4. Consider extracorporeal membrane oxygenation (ECMO), which gives complete respiratory bypass in severe respiratory failure.
5. Correct the hypercapnia and respiratory acidosis through ventilatory support by intubation and mechanical ventilation.
6. Avoid fluid overload.
7. Tracheostomy for acute airway obstruction.
8. Cause-specific treatment

    a. Antibiotics for pneumonia
    b. Thrombolytic drugs
    c. Inhalers
    d. CPAP for chronic failures

Nursing Care Plan

Diagnosis

Impaired Spontaneous Ventilation

1. Acute respiratory failure
2. Altered O2/CO2 levels
3. Breathing muscle fatigue

Evidence

1. Diminished oxygen saturation (< 90%)
2. Diminished PaO2
3. Raised PaCO2
4. Dyspnea/apnea
5. Tachycardia
6. Agitation

Assessment

1. Discuss the patient's care targets.
2. Monitor alterations in consciousness levels.

3. Assess the patient's comfort and amenability when on mechanical ventilation.

Interventions

1. Noninvasive (COPD) intubation/invasive (apnea, respiratory muscle fatigue, alterations in mental status, or worsening acidosis)/intubation with mechanical ventilation.
2. Effective communication with ventilated patient.
3. Prevent ventilator-associated events (VAE) like aspiration pneumonia, pulmonary embolism, and sepsis. Elevate the head of the bed by 30-45 degrees, suction PRN (pro re nata: as the situation demands), reposition the patient, and wash the hands before patient care.

Desired Outcome

1. Patients will have normal ABGs, oxygen saturation > 90%, and reduced dyspnea.
2. Patients will successfully wean off from the ventilator.

Ineffective Airway Clearance

1. Disease exacerbation (COPD, asthma)
2. Neuromuscular dysfunction (myasthenia gravis, ALS, etc.)
3. Excessive mucus
4. Airway spasm
5. Infections
6. Foreign body

Evidence

1. Adventitious/reduced breath sounds
2. Respiratory rhythm changes
3. Dyspnea
4. Cyanosis
5. Copious sputum
6. Weak cough

7. Nasal flaring
8. Agitation

Assessment

1. Assess breath sounds

   a. Wheezing: narrowed/obstructed airways
   b. Crackles and rales: fluid/mucus accumulation

2. Assess respiratory status.
3. Identify patients with risk factors: COPD, cystic fibrosis, difficulty swallowing/coughing (stroke), developmental delays, and muscular dystrophy.

Interventions

1. A sputum sample: identify the cause of the infection and ideal antibiotics.
2. Respiratory devices such as an incentive spirometer or flutter valve can mobilize secretions.
3. Administer bronchodilators to open airways, loosen secretions, and thin mucus, facilitating cough.
4. Suction as necessary.

   a. Suctioning PRN for patients who fail to clear oral secretions.
   b. Tracheostomy requires frequent suctioning.

Desired Outcome

1. Clear airway and adequate cough reflexes.
2. Clear lung auscultation proves effective airway clearance.

Ineffective Breathing Pattern

When breathing is inadequate, oxygenation suffers. Abnormal respiratory rates, respiratory muscle and neuromuscular fatigue, and ventilation-perfusion mismatch can cause respiratory failure.

Evidence

1. Breathing shortness/ shallow/pursed-lip breathing
2. Dyspnea
3. Orthopnea
4. Tachypnea
5. Bradypnea
6. Abnormal chest movements
7. Use of accessory muscle (nasal flares)
8. Cyanosis

Assessment

1. Assess respiratory status; rapid, slow, irregular, shallow, or fatigued breathing indicates ensuing respiratory failure.
2. Assess respiratory history: COPD, emphysema, or chronic bronchitis impair effective breathing.
3. Observe for nasal flaring/grunting: signs of compensatory exertion.

Interventions

1. Check oxygen saturation (oxygenation) and ABGs (systemic acidosis).
2. Apply supplemental oxygen to obtain oxygen saturation levels of 90–94%.
3. Consider noninvasive positive pressure ventilation (NPPV) for COPD (recommended) to open the airways via a mask over the nose and/or mouth with mild air pressure.
4. Administer beta-adrenergic agonists for bronchodilation and corticosteroids to reduce inflammation per prescriptions.
5. Allow rest periods before and after activities to help conserve energy.

Desired Outcome

1. Patients will breathe well with normal ABGs and SpO_2.
2. Patients will not report breathlessness.
3. Patients will cope appropriately.

Pneumonia

Pneumonia is the sixth leading cause of mortality in the US. It occurs due to droplet/contact spread of bacteria or viruses.

Type

1. Community-acquired pneumonia (CAP)
2. Healthcare-associated pneumonia (HCAP) distinguishes patients at higher risks for multidrug-resistant pathogens than CAP

    a. Pneumonia in immunocompromised hosts
    b. Aspiration pneumonia

3. Hospital-acquired pneumonia (HAP)
4. Ventilator-associated pneumonia (VAP)

Nursing Care Plan

1. Assessing the patient's medical history
2. Making a respiratory assessment every four hours, routine physical checks, and ABG measurements

Assessment

1. Cough
2. Sputum production
3. Pleuritic chest pain
4. Shaking chills
5. Fast and shallow breathing
6. Fever

Interventions

1. Maintain airway patency

   a. Check sputum color, viscosity, and smell for changes.

   b. Airway resistance and infection may increase with discolored, persistent, or odorous sputum.

   c. Assess patient hydration; dehydration and thick secretions impede airway clearance.

   d. Frequent position changes and bedhead elevation enhance chest expansion, aeration, and expectoration.

   e. Suctioning can cause hypoxia; hyperoxygenate before, during, and after.

   f. Fluids: 3000 ml/day unless contraindicated (heart failure); warm oral fluids help expectorate secretions. Hydration improves ciliary activity, reduces secretions, and reduces viscosity. Easy to cough up thinner secretions.

   g. Use oxygen or bedside humidifiers.

   h. Assess nebulizer and respiratory physiotherapy effects using incentive spirometer, IPPB, percussion, and postural drainage. Use treatments at least an hour before meals and limit fluids as needed (Vera, 2024).

2. Facilitate gas exchange.
3. Help with breathing exercises and efficacious breathing patterns.
4. Administer correct doses of prescribed medications promptly.
5. Establish infection control mechanisms.
6. Restrict visitors.
7. Institute appropriate isolation protocols.
8. Manage acute pain.
9. Promote rest and graded exercise.
10. Maintain strict bedside and patient hygiene. Provide a covered container for sputum collection.
11. Watch for complications.

   a. Empyema

   b. Hypoxemia/respiratory failure

   c. Pleural effusion

   d. Bacteremia

   e. Delirium (The Confusion Assessment Method (CAM) is a popular screening tool to monitor pneumonia-induced delirium and cognitive abnormalities.)

12. Educate the patient and their families.

Desired Outcome

1. Patients with acceptable ABGs will have enhanced tissue ventilation, oxygenation, and no respiratory discomfort.
2. Patients will optimize gas exchange.
3. Patients will engage in improving oxygenation.
4. Patients will cleanse their airways.
5. The airway will be patent with clear breath sounds, without dyspnea, cyanosis, and secretions.

Thoracic Surgery

Pneumonectomy

Perioperative Guidelines

1. Spirometry: (forced expiratory volume in one second) FEV1 < 80% of normal predicts complications.
2. Actual diffusing capacity: (diffusing capacity of the lungs for carbon monoxide) DLCO < 80% of normal predicts complications.
3. Postoperative FEV1 (calculated) and DLCO (calculated) < 30% of predicted increased mortality risk.
4. Perioperative ABG values are less useful.
5. Exercise testing for marginal patients involves stair-climbing, the shuttle test, integrated cardiopulmonary exercise testing (which measures VO2), and the "six-minute walk test."

Postoperative Management

1. Early extubation and avoiding reintubation

   a. Oxygen supplementation
   b. Shun positive pressure ventilation

2. Chest drains without suction
3. Strict monitoring

4. Sophisticated and multimodal analgesia

    a. Regional block (paravertebral over thoracic epidural)
    b. Opiates
    c. Opiate-sparing agents (NSAIDs and paracetamol)
    d. Ketamine and neuropathic pain management agents (gabapentin, tricyclic antidepressants, etc.)

5. The changes in pulmonary circulation that can cause pulmonary edema

    a. Increased afterload by 50–60% by the right heart
    b. Increased pressure by 50–60% in the pulmonary veins
    c. Increased pressure can cause capillary damage and leakiness
    d. Keep fluid balance as neutral or negative as possible

6. Nasogastric (NG) tube placement is on free drainage
7. Right pneumonectomy patients may develop respiratory problems with gastric distension due to pressure on the remaining lung
8. Left pneumonectomy patients may be allowed earlier feeds
9. Early mobilization

Causes of a distressed patient with a silent chest and the mediastinum shifted toward the silence.

1. Right bronchial tube
2. Main bronchus obstruction

    a. Sputum plugs
    b. Foreign body
    c. Migrated tracheal/bronchial stent
    d. Large blood clot (massive hemoptysis)
    e. Tumor

3. Post pneumonectomy patient with left chest drain on suction.
4. Phrenic nerve damage with a paralyzed hemidiaphragm (Yartsev, 2024).

Nursing Actions

ABG Interpretation

Arterial blood gasses (typically the radial or brachial) assess acid-base balance by measuring arterial blood pH, oxygen, and carbon dioxide.

Values

1. pH: 7.35–7.45
2. PaCO2: 35–45
3. (Bicarbonate) HCO3: 22–26
4. A pH of 7.35–7.39 is slight acidosis, but your interpretation should be "normal."
5. Normal also includes the slightly alkalosis pH 7.41 to 7.45.
6. Acidosis: pH < 7.35.
7. Alkalosis: pH > 7.45.
8. PaCO2 < 35 is alkalosis.
9. PaCO2 > 45 is acidosis.
10. PaCO2 35–45 is in normal range.
11. If *pH and PaCO2 are both* in the acidic/alkaline ranges, the condition is *respiratory acidosis/alkalosis.*
12. If *pH and HCO3 are both* in the acidic/alkaline ranges, the condition is *metabolic acidosis/alkalosis.*
13. If pH is normal, interpret whether it is leaning toward acidosis/alkalosis. Consider other values as well.
14. If pH is normal, it is fully compensated.
15. If all three values are abnormal, they are partially compensated.
16. If PaCO2 or HCO3 is normal and the other is abnormal, it is uncompensated.

Maintain Airway

Several procedures have already been discussed. Some others include:

1. Help the client breathe properly (take a deep breath, hold for two seconds, cough twice or thrice).
2. Utilize a high-frequency chest wall oscillation (HFCWO) vest to clear mucus and bronchial secretions.
3. Failure to cough due to weakness, thick mucus plugs, or excessive production necessitates suctioning. Adventitious breath sounds or secretions require tracheal suctioning. Over-suctioning can induce bronchospasm and damage to tracheal mucosa.

    a. Explain the procedure.
    b. Use lubricated curved-tip soft catheters.
    c. Tell the patient to breathe deeply before and after nasotracheal suctioning.
    d. If the client develops bradycardia, ventricular ectopy, or severe desaturation, stop suctioning and deliver oxygen.
    e. Use Gloves, goggles, and masks (universal protection).

4. Use bronchoscopy for severe problems.
5. Use only prescribed chest physical therapy to mobilize bronchial secretions.

Pre- and Post-Procedural Management

Bronchoscopy

Pre-procedure

1. Check the order.
2. Identify the patient.
3. Ask the patient to remove any clothing, jewelry, etc.
4. Take informed consent.
5. Obtain drug history and allergies.

6. Check for NPO (nothing per mouth) status (6–12 hours before the procedure).
7. Watch vital signs.
8. Instruct oral hygiene.
9. Explain the procedure, interventionists, and the prescribed preoperative medications before giving them.
10. Prepare the patient for local anesthesia.
11. Reassure the patient.
12. Arrange emergency resuscitation equipment at hand.

During the Procedure

1. Position the patient in a sitting or supine position; provide supplemental oxygen as instructed.
2. Assist with the procedure and tissue sampling.
3. Send the labeled specimen to the laboratory directly.
4. Document

    a. Primary care provider's name
    b. Date
    c. Time
    d. Fluid amount, color, and clarity
    e. Nursing assessments and actions

Post-procedure

1. Assess bleeding.
2. Evaluate respiratory status.
3. Monitor vitals.
4. Position the conscious patient in a semi-Fowler's position and an unconscious patient on one side with the head end slightly elevated.
5. Prevent aspiration.
6. Provide reassurance.
7. Offer lozenges/soothing liquid gargle to relieve pain until the gag reflex recovers.

Chest Tube

1. Record a complete pulmonary assessment every two hours.
2. Check the dressing for discharge.
3. Maintain tubing without kinks/occlusions.
4. Monitor water levels in the water-seal and suction-control chambers and add water as needed. Water rises during spontaneous inspiration and falls during expiration. It is absent in

   a. Positive-pressure mechanical ventilation
   b. Kinked/ clamped tubing.
   c. Fully expanded lungs
   d. Mediastinal tubes

5. Intermittent bubbling, correlating to water-seal chamber respirations, shows a pleural space air leak; it will subside with lung expansion. If the water-seal chamber bubbles continuously, check for system leaks.
6. Record drainage amounts and characteristics on the clinical flow sheet every 8 hours.
7. Coughing, deep breathing, and frequent position changes expand the lungs and drain fluids.
8. Removal requires sterile gloves, goggles, a gown, a mask, dressing supplies, a suture-removal kit, rubber-tipped hemostats, and wide occlusive tape.
9. Put the patient in the semi-Fowler posture and put a pad under the site to catch drainage.
10. Instruct the patient to perform the Valsalva technique while the practitioner removes the tube at maximum inspiration.
11. Tape an occlusive dressing to the site immediately after tube removal.

Thoracentesis

Thoracentesis, also known as pleural fluid analysis, involves inserting a needle through the back of the chest wall into the pleural space to extract fluid or air.

All the steps are identical to bronchoscopy, the differences being:

1. NPO may not be necessary.

2. Note if the patient might undergo a diagnostic test to help the doctor locate the fluid.
3. During the procedure, sit the patient on an overbed table with arms lifted. If the patient cannot sit, they can lie sideways on the bed on the unaffected side.
4. Post-procedure, the client should rest on the unaffected side with the head of the bed elevated 30 degrees for at least 30 minutes.

Tracheostomy

Equipment

1. Sterile/disposable tracheostomy cleaning kit/supplies
2. Suction catheter kit
3. Normal saline
4. Gloves
5. Towels
6. Moisture-proof bag
7. Tracheostomy dressing/sterile gauze dressing
8. Twill/velcro ties
9. Sterilized scissors

Procedure

1. The patient is in the semi-Fowler/Fowler position.
2. When opening the tracheostomy kit/sterile goods, be aseptic.
3. Keep the soaking solution and normal sterile saline separate.
4. Suction the entire tracheostomy tube to clear airways.

   a. Rinse the suction catheter.
   b. Unlock the inner cannula.
   c. Remove the dirty dressing.
   d. Peel the glove off, the inside turning out over the dressing.
   e. Discard the dressing and the glove.
   f. Put on sterile gloves.

5. Rinse the inner cannula with sterile normal saline.

6. Replace and secure the inner cannula.
7. Use sterile gauze and normal saline to clean the incision and tube flange. Use half-strength hydrogen peroxide and sterile normal saline to clear crusty secretions.
8. Take dry gauze squares to dry the patient's skin and tube flanges.
9. Place a sterile commercial tracheostomy/V-shaped 4 x 4-inch gauze bandage under the tube flange. Support the tracheostomy tube.
10. Changing tracheostomy ties keeps skin dry and clean. Put tape over the tie knot and a folded 4 x 4-inch gauze square under it. Check the tube location and tracheostomy tie tension routinely.

Home Care

1. Before tracheostomy, wash hands.
2. Explain component functions.
3. How to remove, modify, or replace the inner cannula.
4. Clean the inner cannula two to three times daily.
5. Clean the tracheostomy stoma.
6. Suction if necessary.
7. Check for infection.

End-tidal CO2 (ETco2) Monitoring (Ventilation Vital Sign)

End-tidal carbon dioxide (ETco2) monitoring/capnometry/capnography is a noninvasive technique providing a breath-by-breath analysis and a continuous recording of ventilation.

Benefits

1. Early warning of respiratory compromise.
2. Effective chest compressions in cardiac arrest.
3. Endotracheal tube placement/dislodgement during transport. A sustained ETCO2 level greater than 30 mm Hg for at least three breaths can confirm endotracheal placement.
4. Ventilator circuit integrity is maintained.
5. Earliest indicators of airway compromise during procedural sedation and analgesia (PSA) are possible.
6. During cardiopulmonary resuscitation (CPR), chest compressions should

produce a CO of 17% to 27%, and circulation of CO_2 for exhalation. Since $ETco_2$ and coronary artery perfusion pressures have a linear correlation $ETco_2$ monitoring measures coronary artery blood flow and return of spontaneous circulation during CPR noninvasively.

7. Consuming a bicarbonate solution or carbonated beverage before intubation could alter $ETCO_2$ readings. Capnography is limited in pulseless patients (no CO). It can guide chest compressions—a sudden increase in $ETCO_2$ may indicate restoration of spontaneous circulation.

Pulse Oximeter

The pulse oximeter detects changes in hemoglobin oxygenation saturation and heart rate noninvasively. It uses spectrophotometry and photoplethysmography to determine the percentage of hemoglobin oxygen saturation. The pulsations occurring with each heartbeat are recorded as arterial blood and thus provide arterial blood oxygenation (Lopez, 2023).

Limitations

1. Carbon monoxide poisoning can cause falsely elevated oxygen saturation. Methemoglobinemia results in a falsely low oxygen saturation.
2. Acid-base disorders
3. Low perfusion/hypothermia
4. Severe anemia
5. Methylene blue dye
6. Malpositioning
7. Dark nail polish
8. Excessive motion
9. Ambient light

Quiz

1. What is the effect of fever on an ABG?

    A. The pH will rise
    B. The pH will fall.

C. The pO2 rises.
D. The pCO2 rises.

2.   What is the minimum time by which an ABG sample that is not iced must be tested?

A. Immediately
B. Within 30 minutes
C. One hour
D. Ten minutes

3.   Which is a methylxanthine?

A. Morphine
B. Theophylline
C. Prednisone
D. Atropine

4.   What is the possible imbalance that you would anticipate in a patient admitted three days ago with a tension pneumothorax and prolonged hypoxic state?

A. Hypochloremia
B. Decreased bicarbonate levels
C. Resp alkalosis
D. Hypokalemia

5.   What is the anatomic dead space?

A. Conducting airway
B. Wasted ventilation
C. Minute ventilation
D. End expiratory volume

Answers

1. A. The pH will rise.
2. B. ABG samples that are not iced must be tested within 30 minutes.
3. B. Theophylline is a methylxanthine.
4. A. Chronic respiratory acidosis will allow kidneys to retain bicarbonates and cause hypochloremia.
5. A. The conducting airway where gas exchange doesn't occur.

Chapter Four: Endocrine, Hematological, Neurological, Gastrointestinal, and Renal Problems

Endocrine

Diabetes Mellitus

Types

1. Type 1 diabetes (autoimmune): destruction of the pancreatic beta cells with absolute insulin deficiency.
2. Type 2 diabetes: progressive loss of pancreatic beta cells, insulin resistance, and impaired insulin secretion.
3. Specific types of diabetes: monogenic diabetes syndromes, diseases affecting the exocrine pancreas like cystic fibrosis, and drug-induced diabetes (glucocorticoid) have distinct causes and features.
4. Gestational diabetes mellitus (GDM): diagnosed during the second or third trimester of pregnancy, precipitated by the event.

Values

Values	Prediabetes	Diabetes
HbA1C	5.7–6.4%	≥ 6.5%
Fasting blood sugar (FBS)	100–125 mg/dL	≥ 126 mg/dL
Oral glucose tolerance test (2 hour) 75 g (OGTT)	140–199 mg/dL	≥ 200 mg/dL
Random blood sugar (RBS)	–	≥ 200 mg/dL

Symptoms

1. Polyuria (increased urination)
2. Polydipsia (increased thirst)
3. Polyphagia (increased appetite)
4. Fatigue and listlessness
5. Sudden visual disturbances
6. Premature cataracts
7. Tingling/numbness in feet and hands
8. Dry skin
9. Poorly healing wounds
10. Repeated infections

Interventions

1. Provide patient and family education concerning diagnosis, complications, lifestyle, and follow-ups.
2. Assess and improve coping strategies and skills concerning diabetes self-care.

Diabetic Ketoacidosis (DKA)

DKA is a state of acute insulin deficiency. It typically occurs in Type I diabetes.

Causes

1. Acute infection
2. Missing insulin shots
3. A clogged insulin pump
4. Wrong insulin dose

Features

1. Insulin deficiency resulting in hyperglycemia.
2. Increased lipolysis (breakdown of stored triglycerides) releases free fatty acids that are converted into ketones in the liver as an alternative energy source. Ketones contribute to the metabolic acidosis of DKA.
3. Metabolic acidosis is caused by ketones (acetoacetate, beta-hydroxybutyrate, and acetone). It is compounded by lactic acid due to tissue hypoperfusion resulting from dehydration.

Symptoms

1. Excessive thirst
2. Nausea
3. Abdominal pain
4. Weakness/fatigue
5. Shortness of breath
6. Reports of

   a. Blurry vision
   b. Excessive urination
   c. Vomiting
   d. Fruity-scented breath
   e. Confusion

Signs

1. Hyperglycemia > 400 mg/dL
2. Elevated urine ketone levels
3. Kussmaul breathing
4. Metabolic acidosis with a raised anion gap

Nursing Care Plan

1. Understanding the pathophysiology of DKA
2. Recognizing signs and symptoms of hyperglycemia, ketonemia, acidosis, dehydration, and electrolyte imbalances and assessing them
3. Implementing rapid and effective interventions such as administering insulin, fluid replacement, electrolyte correction, and closely monitoring vital signs and laboratory values
4. Collaborating in multidisciplinary care with physicians, endocrinologists, and dietitians
5. Educating patients on prevention and management, emphasizing the importance of insulin management, regular monitoring, recognizing early signs of DKA, and seeking prompt medical attention when needed

Hyperglycemia

1. FBS > 125 mg/dL
2. Post-prandial blood sugar (PPBS) > 180 mg/dL

Nursing Care Plan

Diagnosis

1. Ineffective health management concerning

   a. Lifestyle
   b. Medication
   c. Glucose monitoring
   d. Stress
   e. Pregnancy

Interventions

1. Instruct

    a. Medication needs (correct dose and time)
    b. Use of glucometers/other equipment
    c. Signs of hypoglycemia
    d. Blood glucose log maintenance
    e. Lifestyle modifications

Hypoglycemia

Hypoglycemia is a fall in blood sugar levels below 70 mg/dL. The brain is the main organ affected.

Symptoms

Of all symptoms, the most common are:

1. Shakiness
2. Sweating
3. Palpitations

Nursing Care Plan

1. In the emergency, start a 50% glucose IV solution/1 mg of glucagon intramuscularly (IM) without IV access in patients with

    a. Seizures
    b. Inability to eat
    c. Very low blood glucose (< 54 mg/dL)

2. Educate

    a. Hypoglycemia can be due to

      i.   Mismatched medications and meal quantity
      ii.   Fasting
      iii.   Heavy exercise on an empty stomach
      iv.   Vomiting/diarrhea leading to poor intake

  b. Frequent testing needs
  c. Symptom recognition
  d. Reinforcing dietary restrictions, including meal times
  e. Prevention and self-management

      i.   Raise blood sugar quickly by having any one of the items below

          1. Small glass of fruit juice/sugary drink (1)
          2. Glucose/dextrose tablets (5)
          3. Large jelly babies (4)
          4. Glucose gel tubes (2)

      ii.   Test your blood sugar after 10–15 minutes.
      iii.   If still below 70 mg/dL, repeat and check after 10 minutes.
      iv.   Eat biscuits, a sandwich, or your next meal to maintain sugar levels.

Hematology

Anemia

Symptomatic anemia: hemoglobin (Hb) < 7.0 g/dL

Normal Hb Values

1. Males: 13.5–18.0 g/dL
2. Females: 12.0–15.0 g/dL
3. Children: 11.0–16.0 g/dL
4. Pregnancy (depends on the trimester) generally > 10.0 g/dL

Classifications

Anemia is classified into the following types depending on the mean corpuscular volume (MCV). Normal MCV is 80–100 fL.

Hypoproliferative Microcytic Anemia (MCV < 80 fl)

1. Iron deficiency anemia
2. Sideroblastic anemia
3. Thalassemia
4. Lead poisoning

Hypoproliferative Normocytic Anemia (MCV 80–100 fL)

1. Anemia of chronic disease (AOCD)
2. Aplastic anemia
3. Multiple myeloma

Hypoproliferative Macrocytic Anemia (MCV > 100 fL)

1. Alcohol
2. Liver disease
3. Hypothyroidism
4. Folate and Vitamin B12 deficiency

Hemolytic Anemia

Hemolytic anemia is a condition in which red blood cells are damaged faster than they are produced, causing anemia.

1. Extravascular: hemoglobinopathies (sickle cell, thalassemias)
2. Intravascular

    a. DIC
    b. Infections
    c. Snakebite

Symptoms

1. Weakness
2. Lethargy
3. Shortness of breath *on exertion*
4. Faintness
5. Pica: eating non-dietary substances
6. Asymptomatic: mild anemia

Signs

1. Cool skin
2. Tachypnea
3. Orthostatic hypotension

Interventions

1. Manage fatigue. Encourage some physical activity and exercise with intervening restful periods to prevent deconditioning.
2. Advise adequate nutrition and restrict alcohol, tea, or caffeinated drinks (interfere with dietary iron absorption).
3. Monitor blood transfusion (vital signs and pulse oximeter) closely.
4. Enhance prescription compliance.
5. Assist patients on high-dose corticosteroids to obtain needed insurance coverage/alternative ways to acquire medication.

Coagulopathies

Impairment of blood clotting leading to prolonged/excessive bleeding following an injury/spontaneously is called coagulopathy.

Drugs

1. Coumadin
2. Platelet inhibitors
3. Heparin

Nursing Care Plan

Assessment

1. Bleeding

   a. Bruising
   b. Petechiae (pinpoint non-blanching spots that measure less than 2 mm)
   c. Hematoma

Diagnosis

1. CBC

   a. Red blood cells
   b. Hb
   c. Hematocrit (Hct)
   d. Platelets

2. Coagulation panel

   a. PT/INR
   b. PTT
   c. Anti-Xa levels

3. Rule of "10": Use the following mnemonics to remember which test is vital for the anticoagulants.

   a. Coumadin *Pt*: 10 letters
   b. Heparin *Ptt*: 10 letters

Interventions

1. Platelet inhibitors: stop; give platelet infusion
2. Coumadin: vitamin K
3. Heparin: protamine sulfate
4. HIT: direct thrombin inhibitor
5. Bleeding: minimize/stop

6. Medication dose/type: adjusted
7. Bleeding signs and symptoms(s/s): advised

Neurology

Encephalopathy

Causes

1. Liver dysfunction (Hepatic Encephalopathy): cirrhosis or acute liver failure with blood ammonia accumulation blood affects the brain.
2. Renal dysfunction (Uremic Encephalopathy): kidney failure causes uremic toxins to accumulate in the bloodstream.
3. Severe infections: viral encephalitis, bacterial meningitis, or septicemia can cause encephalitis.
4. Metabolic disorders: encephalitis can be due to diabetic coma.
5. Toxic substances: medications (opioids/anticonvulsants), chemicals (lead), or environmental toxins (pesticides) can cause encephalitis.

Symptoms

Subjective

1. Mood/personality alterations
2. Affected memory
3. Balance loss
4. Weakness

Objective

1. Altered level of consciousness (LOC)
2. Dysphagia
3. Dysphasia
4. Raised ammonia levels (Hepatic)
5. Decreased thiamine levels and nystagmus (Wernicke's)
6. Shakiness
7. Convulsions

8. Ataxia (abnormal movements)

Nursing Care Plan

Interventions

1. Give specific medications
2. Hepatic: Lactulose (oral/NG/enema)
3. Wernicke's: Thiamine
4. Detailed, frequent neuro exams for LOC changes
5. Perform interventions to minimize intracranial pressure (ICP)
6. Keep HOB 30–45°, note ICP raises in

    a. HOB < 30 = increased blood flow to the brain
    b. HOB > 45 = increased intrathoracic pressure

7. Reduce stimuli
8. Avoid Valsalva techniques (cough)
9. Use seizure precautions (side rails, timely suction, etc.)
10. Monitor respiratory status
11. Consider restraints if agitation/confusion is self-harming

Evaluation

1. Neurological status
2. Laboratory values
3. Seizure activity
4. Fluid and electrolyte balance
5. Patient and family education and feedback

Seizure Disorders

Seizure Activity Phases

1. Prodromal phase with mood/behavior changes preceding seizures by hours/days

2. Aura, visual, auditory, or gustatory, is a premonition of impending seizure activity
3. Ictal stage of seizure activity (musculoskeletal)
4. Postictal stage of confusion/somnolence/irritability

Nursing Care Plan

Diagnosis and Interventions

1. Note the risks for

    a. Injury (muscle)/suffocation (tongue falling back)

       i. Avoid thermometers
       ii. Ensure strict bedrest (prodromal signs/aura)
       iii. Support head, place on the soft area/assist to floor
       iv. Loosen clothing from the neck/chest
       v. Turn the head to one side

    b. Ineffective clearance of airway
    c. Poor self-image related to the stigma
    d. Knowledge insufficiency

       i. Trigger factors
       ii. Medication regimen
       iii. Goodmouth care/regular dental care
       iv. Directions for a missed dose

Stroke

Strokes are ischemic or hemorrhagic cerebrovascular accidents (CVA). Both categories cause brain regions to lose blood supply, nutrients, and oxygen, causing neuronal death and neurological impairments.

Causes

1. Hypertension

2. Arteriosclerosis
3. Emboli (atrial fibrillation/rheumatic fever)
4. Clotting disorders/vasculitis/sickle cell anemia in young

Symptoms

1. Numbness (paresthesia)/facial weakness
2. LOC changes
3. Trouble speaking/interpreting speech
4. Visual disturbances
5. Homonymous hemianopsia (loss of half of the visual field)
6. Peripheral vision
7. Hemiparesis/hemiplegia (weakness/paralysis of the body on one side)
8. Ataxia
9. Dysarthria (articulation problem)
10. Dysphagia (swallowing problem)
11. Expressive aphasia (speaking understandable words loss)
12. Receptive aphasia (comprehending the spoken word loss)

Nursing Care Plan

Assessment

1. Neurologic examinations
2. Vitals
3. Cardiac rhythm
4. Ability to consume
5. Ability to pass urine
6. Muscle force and mobility
7. Mood and demeanor

Interventions

1. Evaluate vitals, mental status, neurological deficits, and LOC frequently and serially.
2. Estimate and monitor pupil size.
3. Evaluate breathing.

4. Evaluate higher functions (speech/memory/cognition).
5. Provide a quiet environment.
6. Raise HOB and bed rails.
7. Leave the nurse bell button at the side of the bed.
8. Control constipation and straining with stool softeners.
9. Watch for convulsions.
10. Provide DVT prophylaxis.

Gastrointestinal (GI)

Functional GI Disorders

Causes

Nutritional losses	Vomiting, nasogastric aspiration, diarrhea, wound drainage, fistula, hemorrhage, ascites, high stoma output
High requirements	Inflammation and infection, malignant disease, growth
Absorption problems	Motility disorders like ileus, extensive disease or resection (reduced absorptive surface), elevated small-bowel transit times, villous atrophy, drugs, and small bowel bacterial overgrowth
Digestive issues	Decreased gastric acid, bile salts, pancreatic and small bowel enzyme secretions
Ingestion	Anorexia, nausea, vomiting, sore mouth, dysphagia, poor dentition, stress, depression, pain, taste perception alterations; can be related to therapeutic/self-imposed dietary modifications

Nursing Care Plan

Assessment

1. History of diet changes. Patients often alter their diet to alleviate symptoms or due to advocacy from non-experts, leading to nutritional deficiencies. Maintain sensitivity when discussing these subjects to avoid criticizing the sufferer.

2. Monitor gastrointestinal losses' frequency, volume, and type to assess therapy response and identify deficiencies.

Digestive Juice Sodium and Potassium Content

Digestive Juice	Sodium	Potassium
Gastric	60	15
Pancreatic	140	5
Bile	145	5
Ileostomy effluent	115	8
Diarrhea	120	25

Interventions

1. Nutritional maintenance

    a. Disease treatment and symptom relief must not harm nutrition.
    b. Doctors, nurses, nutritionists, and pharmacists share expertise. Avoid assuming other professions are aware of difficulties like lesser nutritional intake, muscle loss, poor stamina, and slow wound healing that are apparent during nursing care. Effective communication is key.
    c. Unless therapeutic, do not cut fat if food intake is low. Fats have twice as many calories per gram as carbs or protein, adding taste. Pancreatic and liver disease patients should avoid alcohol since it induces reflux and gastritis.
    d. Patients with GERD should stand during and after meals. Avoid huge meals.
    e. Ulcerative colitis, Crohn's disease, and radiation can produce diarrhea and abdominal pain that stops meals. Provide a snack or liquid food supplement after relaxation and recovery to replenish lost food. This regulation should apply to other underfed patients.

2. Controlling symptoms

    a. Consuming fiber reduces colorectal cancer risk. Irritable bowel syndrome (IBS) requires more. Wind may worsen pain or social discomfort. Make sure consumption creates manageable symptoms.

3. Nutritional replacement

   a. The intestines absorb most salt. Ileostomies require salt in cooking and eating. High ileostomy losses or diarrhea from an intact colon may require oral electrolyte fluid rehydration after limited meal intake.
   b. Vitamin B injections every three months are required for limited absorption in stomach acid insufficiency, resection, and terminal ileum disease.
   c. Fluid loss from wounds, entero-cutaneous fistula, and diarrhea can deplete protein, iron, zinc, water, and electrolytes, necessitating *oral/enteral/parenteral supplementation*. Insufficient nourishment may necessitate a supplement.

4. Depending on the type and quantity of enteral meals consumed, low intake may require *enteral tube feeding* and vitamin and trace element supplements.
5. Poor small bowel absorption or intestinal rest necessitates *parenteral nutrition*_

GI Bleeding

Causes

GI bleeding can be due to upper GI conditions from the mouth to the duodenum.

1. Esophagitis
2. Gastritis
3. Peptic ulcer disease
4. Barrett's esophagus (a precancerous condition of changes in esophageal cell lining due to acid reflux)
5. Esophageal varices (dilated esophageal veins due to portal hypertension that may rupture, causing profuse bleeding)
6. Mallory-Weiss Syndrome (tearing of the esophageal wall due to straining)
7. Erosive gastritis
8. Tumors

Lower GI conditions that cause GI bleeding can occur from the distal small intestine and the entire large intestine.

1. Diverticulosis (colon wall outpouchings)
2. Vascular ectasia of stomach vessels
3. Ischemic colitis
4. Infectious colitis
5. Inflammatory bowel disease (IBS)
6. Hemorrhoids (swollen veins in the lower rectum)

Symptoms and Signs

1. Black and tarry stools
2. Hematochezia (maroon blood with stool)
3. Melena (bloody stool)
4. Hematemesis (bloody vomit)
5. Coffee ground vomit
6. Abdominal pain
7. Signs of shock

   a. BP fall/feeble pulse
   b. Tachycardia
   c. Reduced urine output
   d. Fainting/unconsciousness

Nursing Care Plan

Assessments

The following assessments help with prudent interventions:

1. Deficient fluid volume is related to (r/t) blood loss following gastrointestinal bleeding.
2. Assessment of oxygen requirement secondary to deficient blood volume as shown by fatigue.

3. Insufficient knowledge and anxiety r/t the first episode of gastrointestinal bleeding.
4. Acute pain r/t affected stomach lining following gastrointestinal pathology.

Interventions

1. Volume repletion treats hypovolemia, stabilizes low blood pressure, and corrects postural hypotension.
2. Vasopressin in upper GI bleeding causes vasoconstriction and reduces mesenteric blood flow.
3. Administer prescribed medication. Pharmacological treatment includes reducing stomach acid secretion, managing bleeding, and controlling pain. Proton pump inhibitors reduce stomach acid secretion and slow down inflammation. Vitamin K and protamine are antidotes to some anticoagulants. Reversal agents for all anticoagulants are unavailable.
4. IV pain medication as per oral (PO) pain medication can irritate the GI tract.
5. Instruct about non-pharmacological techniques such as guided imagery, distraction, or heat and cold application for controlling pain (GI bleed Nursing Diagnosis & Care Plan, n.d.).

GI Infections

Gastroenteritis, or stomach flu, is a common, self-limiting, but contagious gastrointestinal infection that causes inflammation of the stomach and intestines.

Causes

1. Viruses: Noro/Rota/Adenoviruses are the most common cause of gastroenteritis.
2. Bacteria

   a. Campylobacter
   b. Escherichia coli (E. coli)Sal
   c. monella
   d. Shigella
   e. Staphylococci

3. Parasites

    a. Giardiasis
    b. Amebiasis

Symptoms

1. Nausea
2. Vomiting/Diarrhea
3. Abdominal cramps
4. Chills/Fever

Complications

1. Fluid and electrolyte loss
2. Dehydration, especially in small children and older adults

Nursing Care Plan

Assessment

1. Assessment of stool characteristics based on history of bowel patterns and the onset/frequency/nature of diarrhea
2. Assessment for vomiting and feeding patterns
3. Assessment of associated symptoms, such as fever and signs of dehydration

Diagnosis

1. Infection risks r/t deficient secondary defenses/ insufficient knowledge regarding pathogen exposure.
2. Skin integrity impairment r/t constantly present diarrheal stools.
3. Deficient fluid volume r/t diarrhea.
4. Imbalanced nutrition r/t nutrient malabsorption.
5. Hyperthermia r/t dehydration.
6. Delayed development risks in chronic diarrhea.

Interventions

1. Controlling diarrhea
2. Minimizing infection risk
3. Maintaining healthy skin condition
4. Improving hydration and nutritional intake
5. Eliminating infection transmission

GI Surgeries

Nursing Care Plan

1. Assess the surgical site/drainage systems.
2. Monitor

   a. Vitals
   b. Signs of infection
   c. Intake/output
   d. Dehydration/shock
   e. Nausea/vomiting
   f. Nasogastric (NG) aspirate/vomit/stools

3. Change wound dressing daily or as needed. Apply dressing around drains and tubes to protect the skin. Encourage personal hygiene. Change positions frequently.

Diminished/absent bowel sounds happen during the post-op period. Start oral fluids once bowel sounds return.

Diagnosis

1. Acute pain r/t surgical incision: Administer prescribed pain medications, encourage patients to change position, and assess after 30 minutes.
2. Nutrition imbalance r/t dietary changes: take daily weight, offer high protein and high-calorie diet if prescribed, and avoid foods that cause bloating.

3. Impaired skin integrity: Assess surgical site/drainage. Change wound dressing daily/as needed and emphasize good personal hygiene.
4. Fluid deficiencies r/t surgery: Monitor dehydration signs, intake/output charts, and serum electrolytes, and take daily weight.
5. Constipation r/t surgery: Ensure hydration, change position, administer laxatives if prescribed, and monitor electrolytes.
6. Infection risks r/t surgery/lowered immunity: check vitals, dressings, IV sites, wound white blood cell (WBC) counts regularly, administer prescribed antibiotics, and maintain asepsis.

Hepatic Disorders

Cirrhosis

Hepatitis cirrhosis causes extensive cell death and fibrotic renewal, leading to hepatic insufficiency and impairing metabolism and waste elimination.

Noncirrhotic forms hepatic fibrosis without liver cell destruction, and mild hepatic dysfunction has a better prognosis.

Types

1. Laennec's cirrhosis (30% to 50%) is the most common.
2. Biliary cirrhosis is the second most common (15% to 20%) cirrhotic condition.
3. Postnecrotic cirrhosis
4. Pigment cirrhosis
5. Idiopathic

Risks

1. Excessive alcohol consumption is the most common cause of cirrhosis.
2. Injury or prolonged obstruction in the biliary passage causes biliary cirrhosis.
3. Hepatitis can cause postnecrotic cirrhosis.
4. Hemochromatosis can cause pigment cirrhosis.

5. Right-sided heart failure.

Complications

1. Portal hypertension (elevation of portal vein pressure)
2. Esophageal varices in esophageal submucosa
3. Hepatic encephalopathy with deteriorating mental status and abnormal movements
4. Fluid volume excess (raised CO and diminished peripheral vascular resistance)

Nursing Care Plan

Assessment

1. Bleeding: skin, gums, stools, and vomitus
2. Fluid retention: daily weight checks and abdominal girth measurement
3. Mental status: behavior or personality changes and level of consciousness

Diagnosis

Nursing diagnosis helps in formulating care plan objectives. Diagnostic aspects concerning cirrhosis include the following.

1. Lower fatigue and increased activity participation.
2. Maintain positive nitrogen balance (muscle mass assessment).
3. Meet nutritional requirements.
4. Reduce pressure ulcer development; maintain skin integrity.
5. Reduce injury risks.
6. Express feelings consistent with improvement of body image and self-esteem.
7. Enhance comfort levels.
8. Restore fluid volume.
9. Improve mental status, ensure safety, and coping ability with cognitive and behavioral changes.
10. Improve respiratory quality.

Nutritional Interventions

1. Ensure a nutritious, high-protein diet supplemented by B-complex vitamins and vitamins A, C, and K.
2. Encourage the patient to eat small, frequent meals.
3. Consider patient preferences within prescribed limits.
4. Provide protein supplements, if indicated.
5. Provide nutrients by NG or TPN if patients can't tolerate oral fluids.
6. Provide patients with fatty stools (steatorrhea) with fat-soluble vitamins A, D, and E supplements and give folic acid and iron to prevent anemia.
7. Provide a temporary low-protein diet for patients showing signs of impending or advancing coma.
8. Restrict salt if needed.

Hepatitis

Hepatitis is a generalized liver inflammation. Most cases are self-limiting; approximately 20% of acute hepatitis B and 50% of hepatitis C cases may progress to chronic hepatitis or cirrhosis.

Causes

1. Infection
2. Bacteria
3. Virus (hepatitis A, B, C, D, E, and G)
4. Autoimmune

Nursing Care Plan

The care plan is centered around the following:

1. Reducing the load on the liver
2. Promoting physical well-being
3. Ameliorating skin issues like breakdowns/itching
4. Preventing complications
5. Enhancing coping strategy

6. Educating the patient about the disease process/prognosis/treatment information
7. Addressing nutritional needs r/t

    a. Meal aversion
    b. Altered taste sensation
    c. Abdominal pain

Nutritional Interventions

1. Mouth care before meals
2. Diet plan depending on the disease condition and patient preference
3. Upright position while eating
4. Fruit juices/carbonated beverages/ hard candy throughout the day (easily digested/tolerated and provide extra calories)
5. Dietitian consultation
6. Medications to facilitate intake
7. Antiemetics like metoclopramide 1/2 hour before meals (Prochlorperazine is contraindicated in hepatic disease).
8. Antacids
9. Vitamins and other dietary supplements as prescribed
10. Steroid therapy alone or in combination with azathioprine per order

Portal Hypertension

Portal hypertension features the following:

1. Ascites (fluid in the peritoneal sac)
2. Shifting dullness/fluid wave on abdominal percussion
3. Dilated abdominal vessels radiating from the umbilicus (caput medusae)
4. Enlarged, palpable spleen (splenic congestion)
5. Bruits over the upper abdominal area (esophageal and gastric varicosities)

Nursing Care Plan

1. Administer medications, including diuretics.

2. Assist the doctor with peritoneal fluid removal (paracentesis). Two or more liters may be removed. Observe the patient for vascular collapse.
3. Measure and record abdominal circumference and body weight daily.
4. Take measures to prevent/reduce edema.
5. Elevate the lower extremities and apply a support hose to prevent lower-extremity edema.
6. Administer salt-poor albumin to raise the serum albumin level. It increases serum osmotic pressure. The ascitic fluid enters the bloodstream and is eliminated by the kidneys, reducing edema.

Ischemic Bowel

The bowel receives 20% to 35% of resting cardiac output; significant damage can rapidly develop when it decreases.

Symptoms

1. Complaints of sudden severe abdominal pain in an elderly individual
2. Nausea/vomiting
3. Diarrhea
4. Abdominal cramps
5. H/O

   a. AFib and peripheral vascular disease
   b. Recent splenectomy

Signs

1. Dry mouth
2. Skin tenting
3. Low BP
4. Rapid, weak pulse
5. No bowel sounds
6. Abdominal guarding

Diagnosis

1. Stool is guaiac-positive.
2. WBC count is elevated.
3. The history, symptoms, and signs may indicate bowel ischemia, a medical emergency.
4. A computed tomography angiography (CTA) scan confirms an ischemic bowel.

Nursing Care Plan

1. Nothing by mouth
2. IV normal saline infusion
3. O2 inhalation to increase vascular perfusion
4. An indwelling urinary catheter to monitor output
5. An NG tube to relieve abdominal distention
6. Cardiac monitor
7. Prescribed analgesic

Desired Outcome

1. CTA scan: no severe bowel damage

   a. Bowel rest and hydration

2. Severe bowel damage

   a. Surgery to remove the damaged area
   b. Thrombectomy in the mesenteric artery/vein if needed
   c. Probable stent placement and anticoagulation therapy

The nurse's critical thinking, assessment skills, and knowledge of bowel ischemia can help patients avoid surgery and save lives.

Malnutrition

Malnutrition includes undernutrition (wasting, stunting, underweight), vitamin and mineral deficiencies, overweight, and obesity, as well as diet-related non-communicable diseases (hyperlipidemia, type 2 diabetes, or HTN).

Symptoms

1. General

    a. Parched and scaly skin
    b. Hair loss/breakable nails
    c. Mouth ulcer
    d. Inadequate weight gain
    e. Electrolyte imbalances
    f. Reduced muscle mass
    g. Weakness/altered mental states
    h. Undersized/delayed development

2. Specific r/t the deficiencies of

    a. Iron (pallor)
    b. Iodine (goiter)
    c. Vit D (rickets)
    d. Vit A (night blindness)
    e. Folate (glossitis)
    f. Zinc (dermatitis)

Nursing Care Plan

1. Identify malnutrition risk factors (diarrhea, pregnancy, infection, stress, etc.).
2. Determine supplemental and nutritional intake/eating habits/medical history.
3. Perform physical checkups.
4. Calculate body mass index (BMI); malnutrition is < 18.
5. Assess dehydration (dry skin and poor skin turgor)/acidosis (headache/tachycardia).

Interventions

1. Provide calories and dietary protein recommended by dietitian and correct deficiencies (Wagner, 2023).
2. Treat underlying condition.
3. Consider temporary NG feeding.
4. Instruct weight loss for overweight (BMI 25–29.9) /obesity (BMI ≥ 30).
5. Emphasize treatment adherence.
6. Educate the patient and family on healthy nutrition and body weight maintenance.

Pancreatitis

Pancreatitis is a painful inflammatory condition that prematurely activates pancreatic enzymes, causing autodigestion. Biliary tract disorders and alcohol cause most pancreatitis.

Nursing Care Plan

Assessment

1. Severe abdominal pain in the upper abdomen/radiating to the back
2. Nausea and vomiting
3. Jaundice in obstructive pancreatitis
4. Weight loss/appetite changes
5. Personal/family history of pancreatitis/pancreatic disorders
6. Abdominal tenderness/guarding on palpation
7. Abdominal distension on percussion
8. Signs of dehydration: dry mucous membranes, diminished skin turgor, or reduced urine output
9. Fever
10. Laboratory findings: elevated pancreatic enzymes (amylase and lipase)

Interventions

1. Manage pain and discomfort due to pancreatitis.

2. Monitor and stabilize vitals.
3. Administer IV fluids and maintain hydration.
4. Keep an NPO status and provide necessary nutritional support.
5. Administer appropriate medications for pain and inflammation management.
6. Monitor pancreatic functions.
7. Address complications (infections/pseudocysts).
8. Educate patients regarding dietary modifications and lifestyle changes to prevent future events.

Renal

Acute Kidney Injury (AKI)

Waste builds up in the blood when the kidneys stop filtering, causing acute kidney injury (AKI) or acute renal failure (ARF). Critically ill patients develop this condition in hours or days.

Risk Factors

1. Advanced age
2. In-hospitalized patients
3. Chronic conditions (diabetes/hypertension/liver disease)

Causes

1. Blood flow impairment (blood loss/severe dehydration)
2. Direct kidney injury (glomerulonephritis/medications)
3. Urinary obstruction (stones/tumors)

Nursing Care Plan

1. Administering medications like diuretics, potassium-lowering drugs, and calcium supplements
2. Caring before, during, and after dialysis
3. Addressing knowledge deficiencies r/t the causes and prevention of AKI

Assessment and Interventions

1. Assess and address cardiac output reduction.
2. Consider a urinary catheter, which can quantify urine output accurately. Intensive monitoring of urine output might improve AKI outcomes.
3. Assess fluid retention; administer/restrict fluids as indicated.
4. Maintain 0.5–1.5 mL/kg/hr urine production. Dark urine with > 1.030 specific gravity indicates dehydration. AKI can progress to the oliguric phase during the diuretic phase without fluid intake (Wagner, 2023).
5. Monitor daily weight; sudden weight gain of 0.5 kg/day can indicate fluid retention, as shown by:

   a. Rales and S3 heart sound
   b. Shortness of breath

6. Assess and address electrolyte balance: hyponatremia and hyperkalemia (> 5.0 mEq/L).
7. Assess and address nutrition status: protein-energy wasting, appetite loss, and malnutrition.

Hemodialysis Monitoring

Only Hemodialysis nurses can flush or touch Quinton's catheters.

1. Limit fluid with input/output monitoring.
2. Administer prescribed antihypertensive drugs.
3. Instruct food restrictions (Na, K, protein).
4. Monitor hematocrit-hemoglobin (H&H) (normal: 12–15 g/dl). H&H around eight/nine is a critical threshold. If ordered, administer two units of blood followed by Epogen.
5. Withhold medications one hour before the procedure.
6. Monitor for increased potassium, BUN, and creatinine levels. Creatinine should be around 1.2.

Chronic kidney disease (CKD)

Chronic kidney disease (CKD) or chronic renal failure (CRF) causes irreversible kidney function loss. As the kidneys are adaptable, symptoms don't appear until nephron loss is significant (stage IV onward).

Stages

1. Stage 1: Normal/increased glomerular filtration rate (GFR ≥ 90)
2. Stage 2: Mild drop (GFR 60–89)
3. Stage 3a: Moderate reduction (GFR 45–59)
4. Stage 3b: Moderate decline (GFR 30–44)
5. Stage 4: Severe reduction (GFR 15–29)
6. Stage 5: Kidney failure mandating dialysis (GFR < 15)

Nursing Care Plan

1. Assess general symptoms r/t water, creatinine, and BUN retentions.
2. Identify risk factors r/t aging/family h/o kidney disease/ethnicity.
3. Document medical history r/t diabetes/HTN/kidney diseases/vesico-ureteric reflux.
4. Assess lifestyle r/t smoking/obesity/nephrotoxic substance exposure (mold/arsenic/lead)
5. Review medications.
6. Assess and manage acidosis/fluid and electrolytes/chronic anemia/bone status (Vit D, calcium, and phosphate binders).
7. Advise to stop smoking/NSAIDs; restrict protein.
8. Initiate dialysis.
9. Provide patient education and coping strategies.

Chronic kidney disease ends in end-stage renal disease (ESRD) or kidney failure. Dialysis/kidney transplantation becomes essential.

Electrolyte Imbalances

Causes

1. Vomiting
2. Diarrhea
3. Disproportionate fluid volume
4. Other medical conditions (renal failure, CHF, hypothyroidism)
5. Medications (diuretics)
6. Malnutrition
7. Surgery/Chemotherapy

Types

Sodium

Hyponatremia: A condition of reduced serum sodium level, <135 mEq/L. Symptoms include nausea/vomiting, headache, and confusion.

Hypernatremia: Serum sodium levels are > 145 mEq/L. Symptoms include extreme thirst, exhaustion, and confusion.

Potassium

Hypokalemia: Serum potassium levels are <3.5 mEq/L. Symptoms include constipation, tachycardia, and muscle cramps.

Hyperkalemia: Serum potassium levels are > 5 mEq/L. Symptoms of hyperkalemia are breathing difficulties, tachycardia, and chest pain.

Calcium

Hypocalcemia: Serum total calcium is < 2.12-2.62 mEq/L. Symptoms include muscle spasm, tetany, and numbness. It can cause life-threatening arrhythmias, or seizures. Always check serum albumin levels for serum calcium estimation.

Hypercalcemia: Serum total calcium value is > 2.12-2.62 mEq/L. Lab results of

Vitamin D deficiency, and CKD can show hypercalcemia. Symptoms include nausea, constipation, and fatigue.

Points to Note

1. Infection and electrolyte imbalances can result from poor drain maintenance.
2. The patient gets the necessary electrolytes from a balanced diet.
3. Recognizing the signs and symptoms of electrolyte imbalance may help the family decide when to call a doctor.

Nursing Actions

Insulin Infusion Titration

Effective and safe insulin infusion protocols have the following components:

1. Must mention appropriate glycemic targets.
2. Should indicate implementation threshold.
3. It is nurse-administered and simple to understand.
4. It has clear instructions for blood glucose monitoring and dose titration.
5. It gives titration based on current blood sugar levels and rate of change.
6. It is safe and has incorporated hypoglycemia protocols.
7. It allows effective sugar control with minimal titration.
8. It has a plan for S/C insulin transition.

Blood Products Administration and Monitoring

Packed Red Cells

Transfuse over 2–3 hours; if the patient cannot tolerate the volume over 4 hours, the blood bank may divide the unit into smaller portions and refrigerate them until needed. One packed red cell should increase hemoglobin by 1% and hematocrit by 3%.

Platelets

Administer fast as tolerated (4 units every 30–60 minutes). Platelet counts should rise by 6000 to 10,000/mm3 each unit. However, immunization from previous transfusions, hemorrhage, fever, infection, autoimmune destruction, and hypertension can reduce incremental gains.

Plasma

Albumin or Ringer's lactate is preferable over plasma for volume expansion with the same hepatitis risk as whole blood. Immediately transfuse fresh frozen plasma to prevent the breakdown of coagulation factors.

Albumin

It increases blood volume in hypovolemic shock and albumin in hypoalbuminemia.

Cryoprecipitate

Used to treat hemophilia A, Von Willebrand's disease, DIC, and uremic hemorrhage.

IX factor concentrate

It is used in hemophilia B to *stop bleeding*. The concentrate pooled from many donors, which increases the risk of hepatitis when treating hemophilia B.

Factor VIII concentration

The heat-treated product reduces hepatitis and HIV risk; they are used to treat hemophilia A.

Complex prothrombin

The indications are congenital or acquired factor deficits.

Blood Transfusion (BT)

1. Affirm doctor's order.
2. Inform the patient and explain the procedure.
3. Check for typing and cross-matching.
4. Take and record vitals.
5. Ensure strict asepsis.
6. At least two licensed nurses check the blood transfusion label.
7. Warm blood at room temperature before transfusion (prevents chills).
8. Two nurses affirm patient identification.
9. Use an 18- to 19-gauge needle.
10. Start infusion slowly at 10 drops/min. Stay at the bedside for 15 to 30 minutes.
11. The adverse reaction (usually occurs during the first 15 to 20 minutes) are

    a. Allergic reactions
    b. Fever
    c. Sepsis
    d. Overload

12. Avoid mixing medications with blood transfusion.
13. Administer saline before, during, or after BT. Avoid IV dextrose (hemolysis) (Vera, 2023).
14. Time

    a. Whole blood, packed RBC = four hours
    b. Plasma, platelets, cryoprecipitate, transfuse = 20 minutes

Bedside Dysphagia Screening

1. Have the client cough and use a tongue blade to test for a gag reflex on both sides of the posterior pharyngeal wall. Avoid relying on a gag reaction to decide feeding time. Depressed reflexes increase aspiration risks.
2. Check for coughing or choking when eating and drinking (aspiration). Coughing while resting or between feedings may suggest food regurgitation or saliva aspiration.
3. Observe pharyngeal reflex. To check the pharyngeal reflex, ask the client

to swallow dry while holding three fingers on the external hypo-laryngeal axis and the index finger on the hyoid bone. The middle and ring fingers are on the thyroid notch and cricoid ring. These structures should rise 2–2.5 millimeters during a dry swallow (Speyer et al., 2021).

4. Assess face muscle strength.
5. Check the oral cavity daily for color, lesions, edema, bleeding, exudate, or dryness. Assess the severity of palate, tongue, gum, and lip ulcerations. Consult a doctor or specialist.
6. Look for fungal/bacterial mucosal infections.
7. Assess loose/broken dentures/tobacco use.

NIH Stroke Scale (NIHSS)

The NIH Stroke Scale (NIHSS) diagnoses stroke-related neurologic impairment and severity, aids treatment selection, and predicts patient outcomes (Naureen, 2024). The assessments are:

1. LOC
2. Age and month communication
3. Ability to blink eyes and squeeze hand on command
4. Horizontal extraocular movement
5. Visual fields and facial palsy
6. Bilateral arm motor drift
7. Bilateral leg motor drift
8. Limb ataxia
9. Sensation
10. Language aphasia
11. Dysarthria
12. Extinction/inattention

Each component scores 0–4, with 0 indicating normal functioning and 4 indicating full impairment. The highest rating after adding up is 42. Higher scores indicate more impairment.

Fecal Containment Devices

Bowel (fecal) incontinence is the inability to control bowel movements due to structural/neurological damage. Stools leak abruptly from the rectum.

Select fecal collection or bowel management systems that collect and dispose of stool. The benefits are:

1. Perianal skin protection
2. Patient protection from C. difficile cross-contamination.
3. Preserved self-esteem

The devices include:

1. The *external anal pouch* has a flexible wafer and a central opening. One side of the wafer attaches to the anal skin and the other to a collection bag. A properly fitted device can last 24 hours.
2. *Intra-anal stool bag* is placed inside the anus and secured with a 10 cm adhesive attachment.
3. *Catheters and rectal tubes* are inserted into the rectum to collect loose stools directly. A water/saline-filled balloon is inflated to secure the tubes.
4. *Rectal trumpets* may reduce rectum lining damage and incontinence-associated dermatitis and improve care. However, rectal hemorrhage can occur.

Drainage and Tube Systems

Drainage tubes (JP, Hemovacs, Penrose, T-tube, percutaneous drains, Foley catheters, nephrostomy) and feeding tubes (NG, nasojejunal (NJ), percutaneous endoscopic gastrostomy (PEG), and PEJ) are used for specific purposes. Know the tube's purpose and location to understand its functions and problems.

Nursing Practice

1. Attach tubes to the skin with a tape (non-allergenic)/device.
2. Secure drainage bags without tension to appropriate locations.
3. Connect the tube to the sterile container. Avoid clamping unless ordered.

4. Ensure the tubing is not kinked or obstructed.
5. Practice strict asepsis around tubes/drainage.
6. Avoid cutting dressings around tubes to prevent wound irritation by frayed fibers.
7. Document and report tube patency and discharge characteristics. Report any spilled amount.
8. Seek help if necessary.

Enteral Nutrition

Based on the patient's enteral formula and feeding duration, two major feeding tubes are prepyloric and postpyloric.

1. The prepyloric tubes, suitable for intermittent feeding, finish above the pyloric sphincter.
2. Postpyloric tubes end beyond the pyloric sphincter in the jejunum and are used for continuous feeding for conditions like gastroparesis, acute pancreatitis, excessive vomiting, and recurrent aspiration.

Some complications include aspiration, tube malpositioning or dislodgment, and agitation. To identify these issues, evaluate and closely monitor the patient before and during tube feeding.

1. Check feeding tube integrity before each shift. Verbal patients with dislodged tubes may experience new-onset pain near the insertion site. Check nonverbal patients' vitals and agitation.
2. Assess HR for refeeding syndrome in chronic malnutrition. It can produce abrupt arrhythmias and multisystem malfunction due to the body's response to nourishment.
3. Flush the tube with a specified quantity of water.
4. Monitor bowel sounds and check for distention and rigidity. Patients experiencing fullness or nausea after meals may have greater gastric residual volumes (GRVs).
5. Observe patients for nausea, bloating, and vomiting and alert the provider.

Parenteral Nutrition

Total Parenteral Nutrition (TPN) is feeding critical nutrients through a central venous line. Clients with a 10% weight loss, inability to take oral food or fluids within seven days post-surgery, and hypercatabolic conditions may have TPN therapy. TPN solutions comprise water (30–40 mL/kg/day), energy (30–45 kcal/kg/day), amino acids (1.0–2.0 g/kg/day), essential fatty acids, electrolytes, vitamins, minerals, and trace elements.

Nursing Priorities

1. Calculate and make a TPN solution using the formula.
2. Assess the patient's nutrition and TPN response.
3. Ensure central venous catheter placement and maintenance for TPN.
4. Monitor and manage TPN-related problems (infection and electrolyte abnormalities).
5. Check and manage blood glucose levels.

Nephrotoxic Medications

1. Acetaminophen and aspirin: chronic interstitial nephritis
2. NSAIDs: chronic kidney disease
3. Antidepressants like fluoxetine, amitriptyline, and doxepin: acute kidney injury
4. Lithium
5. Antihistamines (diphenhydramine): acute kidney injury
6. Antimicrobials (aminoglycosides, antifungals, beta-lactams, quinolones, rifampin, and vancomycin): ARF
7. Antiviral medications (acyclovir and ganciclovir)
8. Pentamidine: acute tubular injury
9. Statins: ARF
10. Proton pump inhibitors: acute interstitial nephritis
11. Angiotensin-converting enzyme inhibitors (ACE inhibitors), angiotensin receptor blockers (ARBs), and diuretics (triamterene)
12. Platelet inhibitors (clopidogrel and ticlopidine): thrombotic microangiopathy (small clots that lead to red blood cell damage)
13. Antiretroviral drugs

14. Calcineurin inhibitors
15. Chemotherapeutic agents (cisplatin, interferon-alfa, methotrexate)
16. IV contrast agents for medical imaging: acute tubular necrosis (This type of renal injury is called contrast-induced nephropathy.)
17. Addictive substances (Heroin, cocaine, methamphetamine): ARF
18. Herbal products: chronic interstitial nephritis

Dialyzable Drugs

Drugs that can be removed by dialysis include:

1. Barbiturates
2. Lithium
3. Isoniazid
4. Salicylates
5. Theophylline/Caffeine (both are methylxanthines)
6. Methanol, metformin
7. Ethylene glycol
8. Depakote/dabigatran
9. Carbamazepine

Quiz

1. Which electrolyte imbalances will you anticipate in a patient with tremors, irritability, and difficulty breathing if he has been taking Milk of Magnesia, Pepto-Bismol, and Tums?

    A. Hyperkalemia
    B. Hypophosphatemia
    C. Hypokalemia
    D. Hyperphosphatemia

2.   Which family member's comments by a family member concerning an unresponsive acute shock patient should worry a critical care nurse most if hypotension persists with IV fluid boluses and vasopressors?

A. Joseph contacted me a couple of days ago to say his prednisone was finished, and he couldn't get it filled for a week.
B. Joseph doesn't like the doctor. Therefore, he didn't want to go to the hospital when he was sick a few days ago.
C. Joseph's family is prone to type 2 diabetes.
D. Joseph has latex and shellfish allergies.

3.   Which nursing instruction is most effective for a 17-year-old patient with type 1 diabetes presenting with lethargy and irritability? Her random blood glucose is 510 mg/dL, and her Hb A1C is 7.5%. She mentioned that she gave insulin dosages when she remembered.

A. If you feel tired, give yourself an extra insulin dose to feel better.
B. Your body does not naturally make insulin, so you must monitor and administer your blood sugars daily.
C. Keep glucose tablets if you forget your insulin.
D. Take insulin before exercising.

4.   Which results support suspected hypothyroidism?

A. Raised TSH, decreased T4
B. Raised TSH, high T4
C. Lowered TSH, high T4
D. Diminished TSH, reduced T4

5.   Which is an appropriate instruction for a patient with hypothyroidism who is prescribed levothyroxine? *Select all that apply.*

A. Avoid soy and fiber-containing foods.
B. Take an extra dose if you miss medication.
C. Take levothyroxine 30–60 minutes before meals.
D. You may crush or chew the medication.

Answers

1. B. Hypophosphatemia can happen as an antacid side effect, particularly with excess magnesium.
2. A. Glucocorticoid-induced adrenal insufficiency may occur from abruptly discontinuing long-term corticosteroids, causing adrenal insufficiency, acute shock, and unresponsive hypotension.
3. B. The patient must take insulin injections to control blood sugar as her body is not making it.
4. A. In hypothyroidism, TSH is raised, and T4 is lowered.
5. A. and C. Avoid soy and fiber rich foods with the medication. Levothyroxine must be taken in an empty stomach.

Chapter Five: Musculoskeletal, Multisystem, and Psychosocial

Musculoskeletal

Assessment and interventions of functional musculoskeletal problems such as gait disorders, falls, and immobility include a h/o (history of):

1. Using braces, canes, walkers, or wheelchairs
2. Recalling falls/near falls in the recent past and whether injured or treated
3. Clarifying current mobility concerning daily activities, whether any changes or need for assistance

Most information about function and mobility comes from patient interviewing. Note posture (kyphosis/scoliosis), walking, and limb movement during the physical exam (Musculoskeletal Assessment, 2023).

1. Evaluate gait.
2. Check the spine.
3. Test the range of motion (ROM) of joints.
4. Assess muscle and limb size and symmetry.
5. Check muscular strength.
6. Feel extremities for tenderness.
7. Check functionality and screen for anomalies.

Multisystem

End of Life

There can be two dying scenarios. Sedation and lethargy can cause a coma and death, or it can involve disorientation, restlessness, muscle spasms, seizures, and death.

Pain: Balance analgesia and patient wakefulness. According to the Rule of Double Effect problem, the American Nurses Association and Palliative Care Nurses Association maintain that minimizing pain and suffering is morally permissible in the dying hours, whether it hastens death (Wholihan and Olson, 2017).

Terminal secretions: Death rattle may be distressing and frightening for family members. Anticholinergic medications (dry the secretions) or turning the patient on their side may help. Avoid suctioning.

The stages include actively dying, transitioning, and imminent phases. Offer your support and care throughout helping the family members cope emotionally with the dying process. Death is imminent (within 24 hours) when:

1. Cardiovascular: Cool and mottled extremities; rapid/irregular pulse
2. Musculoskeletal: Inability to move
3. Neurological: Restlessness, hallucinations, stupor
4. Respiratory: Cheyenne-Stokes respirations, death rattle
5. Urine: Decreased/dark-colored

Healthcare-Acquired Infections

Catheter-Associated Urinary Tract Infections (CAUTI)

The CAUTI guidelines (2015) strongly recommend these evidence-based methods to prevent CAUTI (CAUTI Guidelines, 2015).

1. Use catheters according to indications only as long as they are needed. Those at increased risk for CAUTI mortality are women, older people, and individuals with compromised immunity.

2. Avoid using urinary catheters for incontinence management in patients and nursing home residents.
3. Limit urinary catheter use in surgical patients unless necessary.
4. Remove indwelling catheters from operational patients within 24 hours unless further usage is necessary.

Central-Line-Associated Bloodstream Infections (CLABSI)

Guidelines on insertion, care, and maintenance of central lines by the Centers for Disease Control and Prevention and the Infusion Nurses Society are as follows (Conley, 2016):

1. Set up a closed system.
2. Rub access ports with 70% alcohol for at least 15–20 seconds before access.
3. Choose intermittent infusion caps with a luer-lock design to maintain a secure junction.
4. Change hubs or needleless connectors when there is blood/debris within the cap, when removing the cap from the line, before and after blood sampling (greater patient protection), contamination, and according to organization/manufacturer guidelines/practice.

Patients receiving long-term antibiotic therapy/chemotherapy can be on central lines upon discharge. Educating them and their families about caring for the central line and infection prevention is the nurse's responsibility.

Surgical Site Infection (SSI)

Surgical site infections (SSIs) occur within 30 days following surgery without an implant or one year after an implant. Incisional SSIs might affect the skin or subcutaneous tissue (superficial incisional SSIs), fascia or muscle layers (deep incisional SSIs), or organ space SSIs affecting manipulated body parts.

Complications

1. Readmission
2. Prolonged hospital stay
3. Higher costs of treatment

4. Long-term disability
5. Emotional stress for patients and their families
6. Increased risks of mortality

Strategies for preventing SSIs include:

1. Practice double gloving.
2. Use latex-free gloves.
3. Use alcohol-based hand sanitizer before donning non-sterile gloves.
4. Practice hand hygiene before and after contacting patients.
5. Avoid removing hair at the operative site unless it interferes with the operation; do it outside the operation theater.
6. Avoid using razors.
7. Control blood glucose before, during, and after surgery.
8. Maintain normal body temperature.
9. Use recommended prophylactic antibiotics 30 minutes before surgery.
10. Optimize tissue oxygenation with supplemental O2.
11. Choose a wound protector for gastrointestinal and biliary tract surgical incisions.

Infectious Diseases

Influenza

Interventions for influenza include the following steps:

1. Maintain airway patency
2. Maintain breathing efficiency

   a. Chest physiotherapy
   b. Postural drainage
   c. Change position every 2 hours

3. Encourage fluid intake of at least 2 L/day
4. Achieve normal temperature

a. Antipyretics
b. Tepid sponge baths
c. Hypothermia blanket

5. Provide pain relief

a. Analgesics
b. Warm gargle
c. Throat lozenges

6. Educate about vaccines

Multidrug-Resistant Organisms (MDROs)

MDROs are bacteria that cause systemic infection, prolonging hospital stay and increasing patient morbidity and mortality. They are resistant to one or multiple antibiotics and are difficult to eradicate. The critical MDROs are the following:

1. Methicillin-resistant S. aureus (MRSA)
2. Vancomycin-resistant Enterococci (VRE)
3. Carbapenem-resistant Acinetobacter baumannii (CRAB)

Risk Factors

1. Compromised immunity
2. Hospitalized/long-term care facility patients
3. Aging
4. Patients on ventilators
5. Catheter use

Pain

Acute Pain Management

The World Health Organization (WHO) recommends utilizing analgesics to relieve cancer pain using the three-step analgesic ladder guidelines.

1. Step 1 for mild pain (1–3): nonopioid analgesics with or without coanalgesics.
2. Step 2 for moderate pain (4–6): Opioid or opioid-nonopioid combination with or without coanalgesics.
3. Step 3 for severe pain (7–10): Opioid in ATC-scheduled (around-the-clock) amounts

Nursing Care Plan

Interventions

1. Provide pain relief before it worsens.
2. Recognize the client's pain.
3. Offer nonpharmacologic pain management.

   a. Cognitive-behavioral therapy (CBT)

      i. Distraction
      ii. Guided imagery
      iii. Relaxation techniques
      iv. Reiki

4. Cutaneous stimulation

   a. Massage
   b. Acupressure
   c. Heat/cold applications
   d. Immobilization
   e. Transcutaneous Electrical Nerve Stimulation (TENS)

5. Administer pharmacologic pain management as prescribed.

   a. Use a multimodal approach.
   b. Administer analgesia before painful procedures if possible.
   c. Give nursing care at peak analgesic action.
   d. Evaluate for effectiveness and side effects.

Chronic Pain Management

Some pain-relieving measures include:

1. Obtain the patient's pain ratings, timing, triggering events, and best pain relief information; evaluate regularly.
2. Help choose a pain management plan.
3. Choose opioids, nonopioids, or adjuvant analgesics for the patient.
4. Transfer patients smoothly from parenteral to oral or noninvasive routes using an equianalgesic chart.
5. Administer medications and treatments to improve appetite, bowel elimination, and ability to rest and sleep after taking client feedback on them.
6. Get prescriptions for peristaltic stimulants to avoid opioid-induced constipation and adjust analgesic doses.

Palliative Care

1. Palliative care intermingles with care continuum. The interdisciplinary team addresses physical, intellectual, emotional, social, and spiritual needs and encourages patient freedom, information access, and choice.
2. It involves

   a. Physical: Functionality, stamina, exhaustion, rest, nausea, appetite, constipation, and pain
   b. Psychological: Anxiety, depression, distress, fear, and cognition
   c. Social: Financial burden, roles/relationships, and affection
   d. Spiritual: Hope, suffering, the meaning of pain, faith, and divinity

3. Nursing interventions include:

   a. Inspiring the patient's reasons for care
   b. Listening to the patient and their family members
   c. Communicating with the team and supporting the patient's wishes
   d. Managing end-of-life symptoms
   e. Encouraging reminiscing
   f. Facilitatng participation in religious/spiritual practices
   g. Making referrals to chaplains/clergy/other spiritual support

4. Some things cannot be "fixed."

    a. Death is inevitable for all of us.
    b. Anguish over the death of a loved one.
    c. There are no perfect words/interventions; be present.

Pressure Injuries

Constant pressure causes a lack of blood flow and oxygen, resulting in tissue death and pressure ulcers/decubitus ulcers/bedsores. Prevention is the best strategy as these are unresponsive to ordinary wound dressing.

Risk

1. Aging
2. Immobility
3. Inability to express pain
4. Diabetics
5. Vascular disease patients

Interventions

1. Stage pressure ulcers accurately.
2. Determine additional risk factors.
3. Collaborate with wound care experts to provide wound care.
4. Boost nutrition and hydration.
5. Maintain clean and dry skin.
6. Reposition, practice ROM, and manage pain.
7. Obtain wound cultures.
8. Dispense accurate antibiotics.
9. Ensure proper hand hygiene.
10. Secure intact dressings.
11. Educate on infection prevention.

Rhabdomyolysis

Rhabdomyolysis breaks down muscle fibers and releases muscle components into the circulation. Untreated, it can cause ARF.

Causes

1. Heat stroke
2. Severe convulsion
3. Hypokalemia
4. Trauma
5. Overexertion
6. Ischemia

Signs and Symptoms

1. Weakness
2. Tea-colored urine
3. Myalgia

Interventions

1. Manage the underlying cause.
2. Start early fluid resuscitation to restore renal perfusion with normal saline.
3. Correct hyperkalemia.
4. Consider hemodialysis.
5. Manage secondary complications.

Sepsis

1. Monitor vitals.
2. Assess neurological signs.
3. Procure blood, urine, and sputum cultures and antibiotic sensitivity.
4. Check electrolytes, chest x-ray, renal, and liver function.
5. Ensure DVT and pressure sore prophylaxis.
6. Consult nutrition with a dietitian.
7. Ensure oxygenation and ventilation.

8. Optimize fluid transfusion.
9. Measure input and output.
10. Promote hand washing.
11. Restrict visitors.
12. Educate the family regarding septic shock.

Poisoning

Poisoning with drugs or substances depends on the route, whether ingested, inhaled, or topical, dose, and body weight (children).

Causes

1. Beta-blockers: coma/seizures/ventricular tachycardia
2. Calcium channel blockers: hypotension/conduction defects
3. Chloroquine/hydroxychloroquine: coma/cardiovascular collapse
4. Ecstasy and other amphetamines: agitation/hyperthermia
5. Oral hypoglycemics: coma
6. Camphor: rapidly declining conscious state/seizures
7. Corrosives: gastroesophageal injury
8. Hydrocarbon solvents/kerosene /essential oils: altered consciousness/aspiration pneumonia
9. Naphthalene: methemoglobinemia/hemolysis

Interventions

Consider the Airway, Breathing, Circulation (ABCs) of resuscitation

1. Airway: Secure airway
2. Breathing: Ensure breathing
3. Circulation: Establish circulation
4. Check disability

   a. Seizures
   b. Consider drug-induced syndromes (malignant hyperthermia, serotonin syndrome, and neuroleptic malignant syndrome)

    c. Assess and manage glucose levels

5. Address decontamination

    a. Eyes
    b. Skin
    c. Gastrointestinal lavage: Seek toxicologist's opinion

6. Follow guidelines for antidotes

Wounds

Interventions

The main nursing interventions include:

1. Wound disinfection
2. Decontamination from foreign objects
3. Wound debridement
4. Appropriate wound dressing

Neuropsychiatric Interventions

Altered Mental Status

Altered mental states can represent a variety of diseases affecting mental functioning, ranging from mild disorientation to coma. Fundamentally, a patient's level of consciousness and cognition are combined to form their mental status.

Causes

1. Intracranial diseases
2. Systemic illnesses/infections affecting the central nervous system
3. Environmental toxins

4. Drug withdrawal

Nursing Care Plan

Assessment

1. Lowered Glasgow coma scale (GCS)
2. Altered LOC
3. Poor reflexes
4. Alteratered pulse rate
5. Alteratered BP
6. Raised intracranial pressure
7. Behavioral alterations
8. Disturbed psychomotor functioning

Interventions

1. Execute safety measures.
2. Manage drug or alcohol withdrawal.
3. Treat the underlying condition.
4. Reduce stimuli.
5. Control sundowning (confusion and agitation occurring in the late afternoon and continuing into the night).

   a. Maintain a routine.
   b. Ensure daytime lighting.
   c. Limit napping.
   d. Offer familiar items.

6. Discourage polypharmacy.
7. Educate patients about the causes and symptoms of acute onset confusion to check recurrence.
8. Provide adequate home support on discharge.

Delirium

Delirium is an acute and reversible disturbance in consciousness and cognition. Aging, cognitive decline, acute illness, and a fractured neck femur predispose to delirium. Ask if the patients are more confused than usual.

Causes

1. Medical condition
2. Substance intoxication/withdrawal
3. Prescription side effects

Risk Factor Screening

Use the mnemonic DELIRIUM to remember the assessments.

1. **D**ehydration
2. **E**yes/ears
3. **L**imited movements
4. **I**nfection
5. **R**emember pain
6. **I**mpairment of cognition
7. **U**p during the night
8. **M**edications

Nursing Care Plan

Assessment

1. LOC on admission.
2. Regular risk review.
3. Rapid assessment 4 AT to diagnose confused states faster.
4. The underlying cause.

Interventions

1. Manage the cause.
2. Avoid transferring.
3. Reorient to the present location and time.
4. Provide adequate hydration.
5. Encourage using eyeglasses/hearing aids, if needed.
6. Provide familiar objects/stimulating activities.
7. Maintain a calm environment.
8. Encourage family support.

Dementia

Dementia is deteriorating mental cognition that affects memory, decision-making, personality, and ADLs. The progressive condition is not an aging component. Alzheimer's is the most common dementia.

Risks

1. Falls
2. Wandering
3. Agitation
4. Poor medication management
5. Burns and accidents

Interventions

1. Emphasize communication skills by using simple phrases and a calmer tone. Use nonthreatening body language.
2. Make patient spaces safer, familiar, and organized.
3. Place door alarms or assign a night-watch nurse to patients at risk of wandering.
4. Ensure regular drug administration; watch patients take meds.
5. Use fall risk assessments to help patients who need physical aid or supervision.
6. Develop a comprehensive de-escalation training program.

Disruptive Behaviors

Disruptive behaviors include:

1. Oppositional defiant disorder
2. Conduct disorder
3. Antisocial personality disorder
4. Intermittent explosive disorder

Interventions

1. Reducing violence and improving treatment compliance
2. Building self-esteem and coping abilities
3. Promoting socialization
4. Involving clients and families

Psychological Disorders

Psychological disorders include:

1. Anxiety
2. Depression
3. Substance abuse

Anxiety

Pain, nausea, weakness, and dizziness without a cause are somatoform symptoms of anxiety.

Interventions

1. Assess mental states, triggers, situational circumstances, and personal history.
2. Build and sustain trust.
3. Be calm and nonthreatening.

4. Listen to clients.
5. In the acute phase, relocate the client to a quiet environment with minimum stimuli to provide reassurance and comfort.
6. Consider your mental health.

Depression

To diagnose major depressive disorder (MDD), the Diagnostic and Statistical Manual of Mental Disorders, 5th Edition (DSM-V) requires five symptoms. Some of them include:

1. Persistent depression
2. Anhedonia (compulsory)
3. Worthlessness
4. Lethargy
5. Inattention
6. Altered eating habit

Interventions

1. Ensure safety and self-directed violence prevention.
2. Improve therapeutic partnership and support network.
3. Encourage self-care and ADLs.

   a. Bathing/hygiene
   b. Constipation and bowel movement issues
   c. Sleep and nutrition
   d. Medications

4. Offer emotional support to improve self-worth.
5. Start patient education.

Substance Use

An overwhelming desire to consume more drugs at the expense of other activities is drug abuse. Drug dependence is a physical need/addiction to a specific drug.

Interventions

1. Help the patient to accept the reality.
2. Promote coping strategies.
3. Enhance self-esteem.
4. Educate and encourage healthy nutrition.
5. Advise appropriate sexual functions.
6. Provide education on substance-use consequences and information on drug treatment regarding

    a. Alcohol/opioid use.
    b. Nicotine dependence.

7. Administer medications.

Nursing Actions

Progressive Mobility Measures

Mobility means moving independently, easily, rhythmically, and purposefully in the environment.

Muscle Strength Scale

1. No muscle contraction: 0
2. Some muscle contraction (twitchings): 1
3. Active movement with gravity eliminated: 2
4. Active motion against gravity but not against resistance: 3
5. Active motion against gravity and some resistance: 4
6. Active motion against gravity and full resistance: 5

A joint's full ROM is its maximum movement; for instance, the elbow should be able to extend, flex, upturn for supination, and downturn for pronation. Levels of functional ability include:

1. Level 0: Independent concerning mobility
2. Level 1: Needs assistive device
3. Level 2: Needs assistive device and supervised coaching
4. Level 3: requires an assistive device and direct help.
5. Level 4: Depends completely on others for mobility.

Administer and Monitor Procedural Sedation

Medications for procedural sedation include

1. Benzodiazepines

    a. Midazolam
    b. Diazepam

2. Opioids

    a. Fentanyl

3. Anesthetics

    a. Propofol

The American Society of Anesthesiologists (ASA) affirms that taking clear fluids two hours before procedures doesn't increase aspiration risks in healthy adults. A significant concern for sedation is OSA.

Patient categorization for anesthesia most commonly includes the physical status (PS) classification system (Kost, 2019). While non-anesthesia personnel can sedate PS I, PS II, and well-managed PS III, others are reserved for anesthesiologist intervention.

Types of Pressure Injuries and Wounds

Pressure injuries are prevalent on the sacrum, heels, hip trochanter, and ischium, specifically among people with paraplegia. Braden and Norton scales are commonly used to screen at-risk patients (Aboud and Manna, 2023). Pressure ulcers have four stages:

1. Stage 1: cutaneous erythema
2. Stage 2: erythema with partial loss of epidermis and superficial dermis thickness
3. Stage 3: full-thickness ulcer with subcutaneous fat involvement
4. Stage 4: muscle or bone is involved

Types of wounds:

1. Class 1 wounds are clean, without infection/inflammation/systemic involvement and closed.
2. Class 2 wounds are clean-contaminated, without unusual contamination. There can be controllable exposure of respiratory, genital, or urinary tracts.
3. Class 3 wounds are contaminated but fresh, open wounds.
4. Class 4 wounds are dirty and purulent.

Manage Complex Wounds

A complex wound has one of these features:

1. Duration of more than three months
2. Vascular compromise or necrosis
3. Infection and comorbidities that hinder recovery (Labib and Winters, 2023)

Interventions

1. Fast healing requires a moist and clean environment.
2. Wounds with excessive discharge need secretion absorption.
3. A dry wound needs hydration.
4. An infected wound needs appropriate antimicrobial treatment.

5. A wound with necrotic tissue requires debriding.

Dressings

1. Excess exudate

    a. Hydrogel
    b. Hydrocolloid

2. Highly exudating wounds/pressure ulcers/sinus tract/wounds with exposed tendons/infected wounds (daily change)

    a. Alginate
    b. Hydrofiber (partial-thickness burn/graft)

3. Infected wounds

    a. Hydro conductive dressings
    b. Silver dressing with/without hydrofiber
    c. Manuka honey (MRSA/VRE among others)

4. Scar

    a. Silicone dressing

5. Others

    a. Gauze/impregnated gauze
    b. Iodine dressings
    c. Transparent film for surgical wounds/the donor site of skin graft.
    d. Foam dressing for diabetic foot and minor burns. It is not recommended in dry eschar or arterial ulcers.

Delirium Screening Tool

Confusion Assessment Method (CAM) is an established delirium screening tool. Features 1 and 2 must be present with either feature 3 or 4.

Feature 1: Acute onset and fluctuating course. History r/t this feature is primarily obtained from a family member or nurse and is shown by positive responses to the following questions:

- Is there evidence of an acute change in mental status from the patient's baseline?
- Did the (abnormal) behavior fluctuate during the day, that is, tend to come and go, or increase and decrease in severity?

Feature 2: Inattention. This feature is shown by a positive response to the following question:

- Did the patient have difficulty focusing attention, for example, being easily distracted, or having difficulty keeping track of what was being said?

Feature 3: Disorganized thinking. This feature is shown by a positive response to the following question:

- Was the patient's thinking disorganized or incoherent, such as rambling or irrelevant conversation, unclear or illogical flow of ideas, or unpredictable switching from subject to subject?

Feature 4: Altered level of consciousness. This feature is shown by any answer other than "alert" to the following question:

- Overall, how would you rate this patient's level of consciousness? Alert (normal), vigilant (hyperalert), lethargic (drowsy, easily aroused), stupor (difficult to arouse), or coma (unarousable)?

Alcohol Withdrawal Assessment Tool

The Clinical Institute Withdrawal Assessment Alcohol Scale Revised (CIWA-AR) tool helps family physicians diagnose and treat alcohol withdrawal. It measures 10 alcohol withdrawal symptoms by a direct questionnaire method (Sharp, 2024).

1. Disquiet (0–7)
2. Anxiety (0–7)
3. Auditory, visual, and tactile hallucinations (0–7) each
4. Confusional states (0–7)
5. Headaches (0–7)
6. Vomiting/nausea (0–7)
7. Sudden sweating (0–7)
8. Shaking (0–7)

Scoring

1. Mild withdrawal: 8–10
2. Moderate withdrawal: 8–15
3. Severe withdrawal with possibly imminent delirium tremens: > 15

Suicide Prevention Measures

Use screening tools in the emergency department like the Ask Suicide-Screening Questions (ASQ), Manchester Self-Harm Rule, and Risk of Suicide Questionnaire to assess suicide risks in patients. Asking such direct questions, taking family suicide history, and substance usage can help assess suicide risk from 0-10.

1. Assess risks and establish healing relationships.
2. Establish safety protocols.
3. Install crisis interventions.
4. Offer emotional support and help build self-esteem.
5. Promote coping mechanisms.
6. Address hopelessness.

Quiz

1. Which is the likely cause for nausea, vomiting, stomach cramping, increasing eye and skin itching, and generalized erythematous rash in a 33-year-old with an allogeneic stem cell transplant for persistent leukemia three months before admission to the critical care unit?

   A. Influenza
   B. Kaposi sarcoma
   C. Graft vs. host reaction
   D. Relapse of chronic leukemia

2. Which intervention would the nurse recommend for a patient receiving cooled saline bladder irrigations for therapeutic hypothermia if his temperature dropped from 101.3 to 95°F in two hours?

   A. Notify the provider.
   B. Continue irrigation.
   C. Stop irrigation.
   D. Place a warm blanket over the patient.

3. Which of these statements accurately explains palliative care to a critically ill patient and his family?

   A. Palliative care is hospice and end-of-life services.
   B. Palliative care gives emotional support and symptom amelioration for critically ill patients.
   C. Critically ill patients receive palliative care services.
   D. Palliative care substitutes treatment-focused interventions.

4. Which of these symptoms supports the nurse's concern of imminent neurogenic shock in a 54-year-old patient with a fall leading to spinal cord injury?

   A. Temperature 96°F, blood pressure 65/39, heart rate 38, and cold, moist skin

B. Temperature 102.9°F, blood pressure 190/100, heart rate 149, and warm, flushed skin

C. Temperature 96°F, blood pressure 75/40, heart rate 55, and warm, flushed skin

D. Temperature 103.4°F, blood pressure 104/90, heart rate 140, and cold, sticky skin

5. Which antibiotic resistance is demonstrated by *Klebsiella pneumoniae*?

A. Methicillin
B. Vancomycin
C. Tetracycline
D. Carbapenem

Answers

1. C. This patient's symptoms indicate a graft vs. host reaction, which is common after an organ/bone marrow transplantation.
2. B. For therapeutic hypothermia, quick cooling is essential. The temperature should not drop below 89.6F.
3. B. Palliative care aims to provide emotional support and symptom amelioration for critically ill patients.
4. C. Patients with neurogenic shock typically present with low BP, bradycardia, and hypothermia despite having flushed skin.
5. D. Mechanical ventilation, prolonged antibiotic courses, and invasive and indwelling equipment can cause carbapenem-resistant Klebsiella infections.

Chapter Six: Professional Caring and Ethical Practice

Advocacy (Moral Agency)

1. Recognizing a moral issue, ethical actions, and decisions are all aspects of moral agency. When providing patient care, nurses must balance advocacy and care. Ethics in patient care prioritize autonomy, beneficence, fairness, and non-maleficence.
2. Patient autonomy allows people to choose based on their values and beliefs, potentially contradicting healthcare experts' advice. The nurse must respect a patient's refusal of a potentially beneficial treatment.
3. Avoiding mistreatment, minimizing damage, and advancing patient welfare exemplify beneficence. Medical professionals must balance patient benefits and risks. Helping patients with tasks they cannot do, keeping side rails up to prevent falls, etc., are examples of benevolence.
4. Each patient deserves fair and equitable treatment. Justice entails addressing conflicts of interest, such as healthcare insurance disparity.
5. Do no harm first is the abiding principle of patient treatment. Non-maleficence requires nurses to protect patients and is perhaps the hardest principle to follow.

Caring Practices

Being engaged, open, polite, and addressing the patient as a person can help nurses and patients find value in the caring relationship. Self-reflection can help nurses understand healthcare, empathy, and ethical ideals.

Response to Diversity

The AACN aims to:

1. Enhance academic nursing learning opportunities and experiences and thus quality by learning from varied life experiences, viewpoints, and backgrounds.
2. Inspire nurses and other healthcare workers to serve a *diverse American population* to reduce healthcare inequalities.
3. Improve civic preparedness and nursing students' involvement in leading in health care and society.

Diversity encompasses individual, population, and social traits. Diverse academics, students, staff, and administrators thrive in inclusive environments and cultures. Such environments must *purposefully embrace differences*, not just tolerate them. *Equity* is the ability to perceive gaps in resources or knowledge needed to fully engage in society, especially higher education, and overcome hurdles to ensure justice. Equity requires treating everyone equally, without barriers, preconceptions, or prejudices.

Facilitation of Learning

Nursing students must be able to build and improve competencies for safe, ethical, and effective practice and be supported to grow and network. According to the Professional Standards, Revised 2002, nurses must interact, exchange knowledge, and provide direction to colleagues and nursing trainees in new situations (Practice Guideline Supporting Learners, n.d.).

Collaboration

Nursing excellence requires an organizational structure that supports shared governance—nurses at every level participate in decision-making, data transparency, performance benchmarks, and autonomy.

Efficient and professional collaboration can help establish care frameworks prioritizing clinical quality, safety, and patient experience. Collaboration must uphold patient privacy at all levels to satisfy Health Insurance Portability and Accountability Act (HIPAA) criteria.

Systems Thinking

Quality care requires understanding systems-based practice, encompassing organizational structure and macro-, meso-, and microsystem interactions across healthcare settings. Understanding reimbursement and healthcare cost and payment mechanisms is crucial. Assessing patient outcomes must include how local, regional, national, and global institutions, processes, and legislation affect individuals and varied communities. Nurses champion diversity as change agents and leaders.

Synergy Model

Certified nurse practice is centered around patient care under varying circumstances. The AACN Certification Corporation ensures this by adopting the synergy model, which helps to determine how specifically nursing can be tailored to patients' needs. Careful use of words links patient characteristics with nursing to design a fine-tuned and methodical care system.

The eight competencies that comprise the model include:

1. Clinical judgment
2. Advocacy
3. Clinical practices
4. Collaboration
5. Systems thinking

6. Response to diversity
7. Clinical inquiry
8. Facilitation of learning

Collaboration, systems thinking, advocacy, and moral agency in nursing practice pertain to a patient who is *vulnerable, incapable of decision-making and self-care*, and has *inadequate resource availability*. Similarly, *unstable, highly complex,* or *unpredictable* terms can describe an acutely ill patient. Synergy occurs when a patient's requirements and traits match the nurse's expertise.

Clinical Inquiry

Policymaking, clinical care, and organizational operations must involve nurses as valued and dedicated participants. Only then can the profession excel. Nursing inquiries are of three types:

1. Evidence-based practice (EBP) helps clinical decision-making by solving potential problems with excellent scientific data from patient and practitioner experiences.
2. Quality Improvement (QI) enhances healthcare services, systems, and procedures locally (unit, department, organization).
3. Research involves systematic investigations (quantitative, qualitative, or mixed methodologies) to find, produce, or contribute to new information for patient benefit.

General Nursing Actions

Administer and Monitor Medication Response

Types of Dosing

1. A *routine order* continues unless another order cancels it.
2. *PRN* orders are *patient-requested or as-needed orders.*
3. A *standing order, order set, or protocol* allows nurses to use authorized

prescriptions on any patient in specific circumstances without notifying the doctor.

4. A *one-time order* is a prescription for a single dose.
5. A *STAT order* is issued immediately.
6. *Titration instructions* specific to agency policies in critical care allow the nurse to gradually raise or reduce the medicine dose depending on the patient's condition.

Routes

1. Oral (PO): swallowing tablets/capsules
2. Sublingual (SL): putting under-tongue medications
3. Enteral (NG or PEG): delivered via GI tube
4. Rectal (PR): using rectal suppository
5. Inhalation (INH): inhaling medications
6. Intramuscular (IM): injecting into a muscle
7. Subcutaneous: injecting into the fat tissue beneath the skin (an abbreviation is avoided)
8. Transdermal (TD): applying a skin patch

Check the following drug administration rights thrice before administering medications:

1. Right patient
2. Right medication
3. Correct dose
4. Correct time
5. Correct route
6. Accurate documentation

A recent study recommends ten rights, including the right to history and assessment, the appropriate drug interactions, the right to reject, and the right to learning and information (Vera, 2023).

Nursing Process

An interdependent and dynamic five-step nursing method guides client-centered holistic care.

1. Assessment

   a. History
   b. Observations
   c. Physical examination
   d. Diagnostic test

2. Diagnosis

   a. Identify determining features/high-risk factors/problems
   b. Prepare nursing diagnosis statements

      i.   Actual nursing diagnosis statement
      ii. The risk/high-risk nursing diagnosis statement
      iii. A health promotion or wellness nursing diagnosis statement

   c. Determine/obtain orders/directions from collaborative team members

3. Planning

   a. Priority determination
   b. Written outcome
   c. Nursing intervention
   d. Expected therapeutic outcomes
   e. Outcome integration to care plans/critical pathways

4. Implementation

   a. Physical and emotional requirements
   b. Patient safety
   c. Nursing actions

d. Potential complications
e. Ongoing assessment
f. Care and patient response documentation

5. Evaluation

a. Documentation/reviews
b. Referrals/discharge/treatment continuation

Nursing diagnoses use Abraham Maslow's Hierarchy of Needs to prioritize and organize patient-centered care. Physiological and safety needs lay the foundation for physical and emotional health (Toney-Butler and Thayer, 2023).

Quiz

1. An acute coronary syndrome patient must take clopidogrel after receiving two stents during PCI. However, the patient is uninsured. The expert nurse knows about a pharmaceutical company initiative to help such patients. The expert nurse may also work with social services or discharge planners to help the patient with financial aid. What is this an example of?

    A. Systems thinking
    B. Collaboration
    C. caring practices
    D. Advocacy

2. An 89-year-old patient with metastatic cancer is unresponsive. The nephrologist tells the wife that hemodialysis will help this patient. But the wife is doubtful. The expert nurse will work with the doctor to address the prognosis and the wife's reluctance to continue dialysis and find a better solution. What is this an example of?

    A. Caring
    B. Collaboration
    C. Systems thinking
    D. Facilitation of learning

3. The patient may have three significant risk factors for coronary artery disease after PCI with stent deployment. A skilled nurse will ask the patient which risk factor they want to focus on and recommend based on motivation and seriousness, such as smoking is more serious than a sedentary lifestyle. The nurse will discuss cardiac rehab benefits and arrange for rehab professionals to visit the patient before discharge. What is this an example of?

    A. Client advocacy
    B. Ethical behavior
    C. Clinical efficiency
    D. Facilitation of learning

4. The nurse is caring for a patient who is an enthusiast for complementary therapies. Which are complementary therapies? Select all that apply.

    A. Naproxen sodium for arthritis
    B. St. John's Wort for mild depression
    C. Chiropractic treatment for chronic back pain
    D. Managing seizures with ketosis
    E. IV fluids for moderate-to-severe dehydration
    F. Evening meditation

        i.   A, and B.
        ii. B, D, and F
        iii. B, and E
        iv. B, C, D, and F.

5. Which is *not* one of the quality outcome indicators of the AACN Synergy Model?

    A. Improved compliance with discharge plans
    B. Better critical care admission screening
    C. Improved patient and family satisfaction
    D. Lowering of complication rates

Answers

1. A. The nurse is practicing systems thinking.
2. B. The nurse is collaborating.
3. D. This is an example of facilitation of learning.
4. iv. Complementary therapies should complement the prescribed medical intervention and not substitute them.
5. B. The six quality outcomes include:

   a. Patient and family happiness.
   b. Decreased adverse incident rates.
   c. Reduced complication rates.
   d. Commitment to discharge plans.
   e. Reduced mortality rate.
   f. Reduced length of hospital stay.

Section II:
Practice Tests and Answers

Chapter Seven: Practice Test 1

1.   Which is most likely the cause of a systolic murmur at the right sternal border, second intercostal space (ICS)?

A. Aortic insufficiency
B. Aortic stenosis
C. Mitral stenosis
D. Mitral insufficiency

2.   Which compensates VQ shunting (ventilation-perfusion)?

A. Increased CO
B. Bronchoconstriction
C. Reduced MV
D. Pulmonary vasculature contraction

3.   The nurse examines a postoperative patient with open-heart surgery; she fears cardiac tamponade. Which finding contradicts this diagnosis?

A. Muffled cardiac sounds
B. Raised CVP
C. Raised BP
D. Distended neck veins

4. Which diagnosis conforms to the ECG findings of a patient with heart palpitations and chest pain showing HR 200 bpm, slightly narrowed QRS complexes, and overlapping P with prior T waves?

   A. Supraventricular tachycardia
   B. Atrial flutter
   C. Atrial tachycardia
   D. Ventricular fibrillation

5. What should a nurse explain if a patient questions the nurse as to why he is getting Eptifibatide?

   A. Increases vascular resistance
   B. Reduces platelet binding
   C. Reduces coagulation factors
   D. Reduces cardiac preload

6. Which of these complications would the nurse *least* expect in a patient following an endarterectomy procedure?

   A. Hematuria
   B. Hemorrhage
   C. Hyperperfusion syndrome
   D. Headache

7. Which medication is given to reverse warfarin action in a six-day postoperative open cardiac valve replacement patient on warfarin if her INR is 5.2 and she has oozing bloody wound drainage and generalized bruises?

   A. Glucagon
   B. Vitamin K
   C. Naloxone
   D. Protamine

8. Which is the most appropriate interpretation for RR = 40/minute, labored breathing, PaO2 = 68, PaCO2 = 50, pH 7.34, HCO3 = 22, and SaO2 = 91%?

    A. COPD
    B. Upper airways obstruction
    C. Metabolic acidosis
    D. Respiratory acidosis

9. What is the *priority* nursing action for an insulin-dependent patient in the ER with increased, labored respirations, fruity breath odor, and a blood glucose of 776 mg/dL?

    A. Inject insulin glargine 200 units.
    B. Give 15 grams of glucose solution.
    C. Perform an IV access.
    D. Prepare for intubation.

10. Which of the following explains several odd-shaped bruises on the back of an 87-year-old woman from a local long-term care facility?

    A. Incidental bruises requiring no further investigation
    B. Possibility of accidental falls
    C. Possibility of elder abuse
    D. Underlying coagulopathy

11. What is the baseline data for pharmacotherapy?

    A. Nursing algorithm
    B. Lab results
    C. Patient information
    D. Physician prescription

12. What is the *minimum* expected urine output over a 12-hour shift for a 78 kg patient at high risk for SIADH?

    A. It's 1060 mL
    B. Minimally 500 mL
    C. Minimally 468 mL

D. It's 2020 mL

13. Which is *not* an expected lab finding in diabetes insipidus (DI)?

    A. Urine specific gravity 1.030
    B. Urine osmolality 120 mOsm/kg
    C. Random plasma osmolality 294 mOsm/kg
    D. Sodium level 150 mEq/L

14. What is normal urine specific gravity?

    A. <1.005
    B. 1.036
    C. 1.005–1.030
    D. 1.05

15. Which change in ventilator setting can increase CO_2 elimination?

    A. Lowering the frequency
    B. Increasing FiO_2
    C. Increasing the mean airway pressure (Paw)
    D. Lowering power

16. What is the risk factor for hyperglycemic hyperosmolar nonketotic syndrome (HHNK)?

    A. Hypernatremia
    B. Age 20 years
    C. Chronic illness
    D. Furosemide prescription

17. What is a risk factors for falls?

    A. Dementia
    B. Poor nutrition
    C. Shock
    D. Open skin wounds

18. What history is not vital in an insulin-dependent patient in the ER with increased, labored respirations, fruity breath odor, and a blood glucose of 700 mg/dL?

    A. Did he take his insulin regularly?
    B. When was the last meal?
    C. Where did he take his insulin?
    D. Where did he keep his insulin?

19. Which statement suggests the need for better medication education for a newly diagnosed hypertensive patient who receives discharge instructions on atenolol from the nurse?

    A. "If my blood pressure is normal, I can skip atenolol."
    B. "I must take atenolol every day at the same time."
    C. "I must inform my doctor of any medication changes."
    D. "In addition to atenolol, I must consume less sodium and exercise more."

20. Who is at the *highest* risk for hypertensive encephalopathy?

    A. A 48-year-old HTN male who has discontinued his antihypertensive medication.
    B. A 45-year-old woman with anxiety
    C. An 85-year-old male with intracerebral hemorrhage and 180/83 BP.
    D. A 26-year-old woman with delirium tremens

21. Which is not true for paradoxical breathing?

    A. Impending diaphragmatic failure
    B. Happens in children
    C. Airway obstruction
    D. Yoga practice

22. Which grade of hemorrhage is apt for a CCU patient with subarachnoid hemorrhage having confusion and mild focal neurological deficit?

    A. Grade III

B. Grade I

C. Grade V

D. Grade II

23. Which of the following events is most concerning about platelet level of 10,000 cu/mL in acute idiopathic thrombocytopenic purpura (ITP)?

A. Epistaxis

B. Subconjunctival hemorrhage

C. Intracranial hemorrhage

D. Purpura

24. Which platelet count is at a greater risk for intracranial hemorrhage?

A. Count<20,000 cu/mL

B. Count<30,000 cu/mL

C. Count>20,000 cu/mL

D. Count<25, 000 cu/mL

25. Which of these values indicates COPD?

A. FEV1/FVC>80%

B. FEV1/FVC<65%

C. FEV1/FVC 70–80%

D. FEV1/FVC Normal

26. Which is *not* a brain death criterion?

A. No oculovestibular reflex

B. apnea without ventilator aid

C. No oculocephalic reflex

D. Irregular EEG waves

27. Which of the following statements by the patient indicates that he understands why he's having balloon angioplasty for peripheral vascular insufficiency?

A. "This technique compresses blocked arteries to allow blood flow."

B. "This treatment will allow me to live normally without arterial blood flow blockage."

C. "This surgery lowers my stroke risk."

D. "This treatment will open the obstruction without a stent."

28. Which statement is correct in providing more information on erythropoietin to a patient in the ICU?

A. It boosts white blood cell production.
B. It prevents hypotension.
C. It boosts red blood cells.
D. It slows blood coagulation.

29. Which neuromuscular blockade would you anticipate with an ordered 2/4 twitch for a patient who continues to "buck the ventilator"?

A. Blockage: 70%
B. Blockage: 99%
C. Blockage: 90%
D. Blockage: 0–75%

30. Which instruction on preparation allows appropriate administration of tissue plasminogen activator (tPA)?

A. Split 100 mg into 10 mg given over 1 minute and 90 mg administered over 60 minutes.
B. Divide 100 mg into 10 mg over 5 minutes and 91 mg over 30 minutes.
C. Dispense 100 mg into 12 mg over 1 minute and 88 mg over 30 minutes.
D. Split 100 mg into 12 mg over 1 minute and 88 mg administered over 60 minutes.

31. What is the priority intervention in DKA?

A. Fluid resuscitation
B. IV insulin
C. Oxygen supplementation
D. Bicarbonate administration

32. Which of the following instructions would you question for a 63-year-old ER patient with abdominal pain, nausea, and vomiting and no bowel movements for several days?

    A. Strict IO measurements
    B. A PO challenge
    C. Low intermittent gastric suction
    D. Isotonic fluid administration

33. What must a nurse immediately perform on a post-cardiac cath patient if the patient complains of abdominal and back pain and the nurse finds the patient bradycardic and hypotensive?

    A. Administer a 1000 mL IV fluid bolus.
    B. Report the primary physician.
    C. Administer scheduled pain medication.
    D. Pivot the patient on his left side.

34. What is the first-line drug treatment recommended for life-threatening asthma?

    A. Anticholinergic
    B. Leukotriene receptor antagonist
    C. β-selective agonist
    D. Antibiotics

35. What is the least endotracheal tube cuff pressure to prevent aspiration of secretions?

    A. 11 cm H2O
    B. 30 cm H2O
    C. 20 cm H2O
    D. 28 cm H2O

36. Which is a priority when implementing pain evaluation and management strategies?

    A. Patients must know about potential adverse effects.
    B. Care spans across disciplines.
    C. No two people feel pain in the same way.
    D. Pain management depends on the patient's goals.

37. What is the PaO2/FiO2 for a patient admitted in ICU with ARDS with ABG showing PaCO2 48, PaO2 82, pH 7.5, SaO2 94, and ventilator findings PEEP 5, Rate 16 40%, and SIMV 550mL TV?

    A. PaO2/FiO2 = 225
    B. PaO2/FiO2 =205
    C. PaO2/FiO2 = 220
    D. PaO2/FiO2 = 126

38. What is the telemetric diagnosis of a rhythm that shows a gradual PR interval increase until a P wave is blocked and the next QRS complex is dropped?

    A. Second-degree AV block, Type II
    B. Third-degree AV block
    C. Second-degree AV block, Type I
    D. First-degree AV block

39. Which PaO2/FiO2 value indicates acute respiratory failure?

    A. PaO2/FiO2>350
    B. PaO2/FiO2<350
    C. PaO2/FiO2<300
    D. PaO2/FiO2>430

40. What is the *priority* nursing action for a patient immediately after post-operative transcatheter aortic valve replacement who is restless and keels over?

    A. Sedate the patient.

B. Start early ambulation.
C. Reorient to a flat position.
D. Assist to a sitting position.

41.   Which of the following can cause ventilatory abnormalities in a COPD patient on high FiO2 levels?

A. Increased WOB
B. Increased dead space
C. Bronchoconstriction
D. Sputum production

42.   While reviewing the electronic medication record of a patient with a prolonged QT interval, the nurse should question which of these medication orders?

A. Diphenhydramine 50 mg PO six hourly
B. Metformin 500 mg PO twice daily
C. Hydrochlorothiazide 25 mg PO daily
D. Nadolol 40 mg PO daily

43.   Which of these signify ventilator need for a COPD patient?

A. Wheezing inspiration
B. Paradoxical breathing
C. PaCO2 55
D. Purulent sputum

44.   Which is the *most* appropriate response for patient inquiries about an impending femoral-popliteal bypass?

A. "The saphenous vein is typically used to bypass the block."
B. "The mammary vein is typically used to bypass the obstruction."
C. "The saphenous artery is used to bypass the blockage."
D. "The brachial artery is taken to bypass the blockage."

45. What is the *priority* nursing intervention in a 65-year-old male with DVT on s/c heparin with Hgb 13.0 gm/dL, Hct 56%, and platelets 48,000 platelets/mcL?

    A. Give supplemental oxygen via face mask.
    B. Give the scheduled dose of heparin.
    C. Start an IV.
    D. Inform the provider.

46. What is the time of action of sublingual nitroglycerin?

    A. Two seconds
    B. Four minutes
    C. Ten minutes
    D. Fifteen seconds

47. What is the most effective route for bronchodilator administration?

    A. Oral
    B. Suppository
    C. IV
    D. Inhalation

48. Which insulin preparation is used to treat DKA?

    A. Insulin Glargine
    B. NPH
    C. Regular
    D. Aspart

49. Which foods should a nurse instruct a patient with GERD to avoid?

    A. Bananas
    B. White bread
    C. Baked salmon
    D. Tomatoes

50. What does an ABG PaO2/FiO2 84 indicate in a patient on ventilator with wrosening hypoxia?

    A. Mild hypoxia
    B. Severe hypoxia
    C. Moderate hypoxia
    D. Normal value

51. Which of these indicates an acute or chronic respiratory failure in an ICU-admitted COPD patient with a smoking history?

    A. PaO2 60
    B. PaCO2 65
    C. pH 7.3
    D. SaO2 91%

52. Which is a priority nursing intervention if a patient receiving a packed RBC transfusion becomes agitated and tachypneic suddenly?

    A. Give diphenhydramine.
    B. Inform the provider.
    C. Raise infusion rate.
    D. Stop transfusion.

53. Which condition is suspected in a patient complaining of generalized numbness, tingling, and lower limb weakness after an influenza vaccine?

    A. Guillain-Barre′ syndrome
    B. Syringomyelia
    C. Meningitis
    D. Myelitis

54. What cardiac cycle percentage do atrial kicks provide?

    A. Twenty
    B. Thirty
    C. Eighteen
    D. Forty

55. Which statement of the patient during his discharge indicates an understanding of epileptic emergencies?

   A. Status epilepticus is a notifiable medical emergency.
   B. I can avoid status epilepticus with regular medications.
   C. My caregiver may administer an additional dose of my antiepileptics if I have seizures.
   D. I should keep my emergency diazepam at home.

56. Which intervention would you anticipate occurring *last* in Grade 3 splenic injury with 10g/dL Hb and Hct 33?

   A. Infuse a unit of packed RBC.
   B. Prepare for splenic removal.
   C. Perform frequent abdominal assessments.
   D. Place the patient on restricted activity.

57. Which is best to treat auto-PEEP in an agitated patient (breathing rate 20 and assist control (AC) rate 10)?

   A. Administer sedative
   B. Raise flow rate
   C. Use bronchodilators
   D. Reduce TV

58. A patient with CHF has daily weight checks and intake output monitoring. The nurse notes that the client's 24-hour intake and output were 2200 mL and 1200 mL, respectively. What is the expected weight for the next day?

   A. Weight drop of 1 lb
   B. Weight gain of 1.2 lb
   C. Weight loss of 2 lb
   D. Weight gain of 2.2 lb

59. What is compartment syndrome?

   A. Compartmentalizing emotions.

B. Restricting pathogens.

C. Building-up of pressure from internal bleeding

D. Isolating patients

60. Which of these bacteria causes bacterial meningitis?

A. Streptococcus pyogenes

B. E. coli

C. Streptococcus pneumoniae

D. Staphylococcus aureus

61. Which is a priority action if a patient's phenobarbital level is 47 µg/mL?

A. Withhold the next phenobarbital dose.

B. Inform the provider.

C. Give bolus phenobarbital.

D. No intervention.

62. Which indicates phenobarbital toxicity?

A. Blood level >40 µg/mL

B. Blood level >15 µg/mL

C. Blood level>10 µg/mL

D. Blood level>35 µg/mL

63. Which has a narrow therapeutic index?

A. Levothyroxine

B. Paracetamol

C. Cephalosporin

D. Vitamin A

64. What is the first treatment for pulmonary edema?

A. Oxygen inhalation

B. Restrict fluids.

C. Give diuretics

D. Elevate HOB.

65.   Which acute asthma presentation needs ICU management?

    A. Dyspnea affecting ADLs
    B. Inability to complete a sentence
    C. Inspiratory wheezes
    D. Corticosteroid administration

66.   What is the priority intervention for a patient with h/o CAD who has come to the ER with complaints of sudden onset chest pain and profuse sweating?

    A. Give aspirin
    B. Give oxygen
    C. Give morphine
    D. Communicate with the interprofessional team

67.   What is critical evidence-based management for MI?

    A. The prognosis is better with early intervention.
    B. Lab parameters are crucial.
    C. Mortality is lower in females.
    D. PCI is the best treatment modality.

68.   What is the indication for oxygenation in MI?

    A. Routine on admission
    B. Pulse oximetry < 94% (room air)
    C. Pulse oximetry < 98% (room air)
    D. Not needed

69.   Which IV medication can create a transient asystole in treating ventricular tachycardia?

    A. Lidocaine
    B. Adenosine
    C. Adrenaline
    D. Bretylium

70. What is the ventilator-induced shearing injury of the lung called?

    A. Atelectrauma
    B. Barotrauma
    C. Biotrauma
    D. Volutrauma

71. Which indicates a compartment syndrome?

    A. Increased CVP
    B. Increased CO
    C. Increased GFR
    D. None of these

72. What is a normal EF?

    A. 65%
    B. 18%
    C. 25%
    D. 30%

73. What is the CO for a patient with 75 HR and SV of 70 mL?

    A. CO = 5 L/minute
    B. CO = 6 L/minute
    C. CO = 4.4 mL/minute
    D. CO = 5.2 mL/minute

74. Which intervention is indicated for a patient with acute intracranial hemorrhage?

    A. Provide raised HOB position.
    B. Keep patient in Trendelenburg.
    C. Give supplemental oxygen.
    D. Perform nerve stimulation.

75.   Which statement provides the *best* opportunity for de-escalating a patient who is becoming increasingly loud and agitated?

A. Your frustration is evident. What's troubling you?
B. I won't help until you speak like an adult.
C. Please quiet down, or I'll give you PRN Ativan!
D. You must breathe.

76.   Which is the most common test for assessing mobility and balance?

A. Six-minute walk test (6MWT)
B. Ten-minute shuttle walk
C. Up and go test
D. Functional reach test

77.   Which would be *inappropriate* action for an ICU patient with a sudden onset of pulmonary edema following CHF exacerbation?

A. Administer morphine every four hours.
B. Withhold scheduled furosemide.
C. Give 100% oxygen via face mask.
D. Position the patient in a high Fowler's position.

78.   Which of these is valid for medicaid plan B?

A. It applies to nurses' charges.
B. Insulin pumps are available.
C. It has a penalty.
D. All of the above.

79.   What is the immediate treatment for AFib?

A. Cardiac ablation
B. Cardiac rehabilitation
C. Patient education
D. Rhythm control

80. Which is the most appropriate advice on discharge for a 35-year-old obese female with OSA?

    A. C-PAP/BiPAP usage
    B. Night-time oximetry monitoring
    C. Daytime sedation reduction
    D. Weight reduction and oxygen via C-PAP/BiPAP

81. Which elevated pulmonary vascular resistance is classified as PAH?

    A. Pulmonary embolism
    B. Idiopathic
    C. LVF
    D. COPD

82. Which of these tests should a nurse anticipate to monitor a continuous heparin infusion to treat DVT?

    A. PT, INR
    B. D-dimer
    C. aPTT, anti-Xa
    D. Troponin, creatinine kinase

83. Which discharge advice plan is appropriate for a 56-year-old patient with DVT?

    A. Oral and written instructions
    B. Verbal instructions
    C. Written instructions
    D. No special instructions are required

84. Which ventilator adjustments can be altered to increase tidal volume (TV)?

    A. Reduce the flow rate
    B. Reduce RR
    C. Raise the PEEP
    D. Raise the pressure limit

85. Which long-term treatment is correct for a 76-year-old patient with asthma with persistent nocturnal wheezing?

    A. Montelukast
    B. B-blockers.
    C. Ipratropium bromide
    D. Inhaled steroids.

86. Which nursing intervention is *most* appropriate for a severely agitated, aggressive, intoxicated patient who is under restraints for his safety?

    A. Diminish triggers around the patient.
    B. Summon a public safety officer.
    C. Attempt patient reorientation and feedback.
    D. Assess physical restraint after every 15 minutes.

87. Which statement by the patient displays an understanding of chlorothiazide precautions?

    A. If I drink more fluids, I can take chlorothiazide.
    B. Getting out of bed quickly will prevent dizziness.
    C. To avoid the effects of the medication, I must eat more salt.
    D. Sunscreen is a must before going out.

88. Which statement best explains Wolff-Parkinson-White (WPW) syndrome to a newly diagnosed patient?

    A. "WPW slows the heart rate."
    B. "WPW is a CVD-related adulthood condition."
    C. "WPW develops in uncontrolled chronic HTN."
    D. "WPW is present at birth."

89. Which assessment finding supports a suspicion of manual strangulation in a domestic dispute?

    A. Peripheral cyanosis of the face
    B. V-shaped marking on the throat
    C. Facial petechiae

D. Ligature markings

90. Which diagnosis should you anticipate if the patient's wife states that the patient has more frequent, severe, and prolonged chest pain than before?

A. Exertional angina
B. Variant angina
C. Stable angina
D. Unstable angina

91. What part of the cardiac cycle is diastole?

A. One-half
B. Two-third
C. One-third
D. One-fourth

92. Which is the *most* appropriate to a patient's query regarding ambulation after a femoral entry interventional cardiac catheterization?

A. "You must lie flat for six hours after your procedure."
B. "You must lie flat for four hours after your procedure."
C. "You will be lying flat for two hours."
D. "Interventional cardiac catheterization doesn't require any fixed post-procedural resting period."

93. Which of these assessments indicates a potential problem for a cardiac pacemaker placement for symptomatic bradycardia?

A. Constant hiccups
B. Insertion-site blood-stained drainage
C. Peripheral capillary refill three seconds
D. HTN

94. Which sign can signify hyperglycemia in gestational diabetes presenting with excessive thirst and hunger?

A. Reduced urination

      B. Blurred vision
      C. Weight gain
      D. Frequent urination

95.   What is the mean arterial pressure (MAP) for a patient with systolic pressure (SP) 130, diastolic pressure (DP) 70, and HR 70?

      A. 80 mm Hg
      B. 90 mmHg
      C. 78 mm Hg
      D. 68 mm Hg

96.   What is the CI (cardiac index) if CO is 5 L/minute and BSA (body surface area) is 1.25 m2?

      A. 3.6 L/min/m2.
      B. 2.5 L/min/m2
      C. 1.8 L/min/m2
      D. 3 L/min/m2

97.   What condition does an ABG with pH 7.31, PaCO2 53 mm Hg, HCO3 24 mm Hg, and SpO2 93% signify?

      A. Compensated respiratory acidosis
      B. Uncompensated respiratory alkalosis
      C. Uncompensated respiratory acidosis
      D. Compensated respiratory alkalosis

98.   Which are the *most* common chemical restraints?

      A. Antiepileptics
      B. Narcotics
      C. Stimulants
      D. Benzodiazepines

99. What should you anticipate if a patient voids foul-odored urine, develops flank pain, fever, chills, and increased urine frequency 48 hours after laser lithotripsy with stent placement?

     A. Surgery recovery
     B. Pyelonephritis
     C. Kidney stone
     D. Acute tubular necrosis

100. Which test would you suggest in a patient with IBD with abdominal pain, fever, and bloody diarrhea?

     A. Barium swallow
     B. Abdominal USG
     C. Colonoscopic biopsy
     D. Stool culture

101. Which is crucial to insulin administration in terms of hypoglycemia prevention?

     A. Inject IM.
     B. Store insulin at room temperature.
     C. Rotate injection sites frequently.
     D. Increase dosages during illness.

102. Why must patients lie flat after a femoral entry cardiac catheterization?

     A. To check internal bleeding only.
     B. To check external bleeding only.
     C. To overcome sedation effects.
     D. To reduce internal and external bleeds.

103. Which of these assessments is most concerning for a DVT in a case of prolonged immobility?

     A. One second capillary refill
     B. Erythema both limbs
     C. Weakness in the immobilized leg

        D. Positive Homan's sign (foot dorsiflexion causes calf pain)

104.   What is the minimum MAP?

        A. 78 mm Hg
        B. 90 mm Hg
        C. 80 mm Hg
        D. 60 mm Hg

105.   What is the appropriate action in a post-aortic aneurysm repair patient with reduced appetite and energy on the second post-op day?

        A. Give an oral antiemetic.
        B. Inform the primary provider.
        C. Administer high-calorie nutritional supplements.
        D. Encourage movements.

106.   What should you do if a 78-year-old patient with h/o hemorrhoids has bright red stools and dizziness?

        A. Start IV.
        B. Elevate lower limbs.
        C. Administer pain relief medicines.
        D. Give IV antibiotics.

107.   What is appropriate if you notice that a patient develops sudden dyspnea and chest pain with diminished breath sounds on the right side 72 hours post-cardiac surgery?

        A. Reposition the patient
        B. Encourage breathing and coughing.
        C. Notify the provider.
        D. Give pain medication.

108.   What percentage of coronary artery blockage can cause angina?

        A. 55%

B. 70%

C. 75%

D. 80%

109. What is a priority in a 75-year-old patient admitted with profuse diarrhea?

   A. Give IV metronidazole
   B. Encourage oral fluids
   C. Assess electrolytes
   D. Initiate enteric precautions

110. What is the priority consideration for effective discharge planning of a retired patient with no insurance who was on observation for chest pain?

   A. Weekly home health care
   B. Arrangement for a 3-month cardiology appointment
   C. Gym membership suggestion
   D. Arrangement for OTC emergency medication

111. What action is appropriate if you notice an increase in chest tube drainage 48 hours post-CABG?

   A. Seek for a blood transfusion order.
   B. Give diuretics.
   C. Encourage breathing exercises.
   D. Assess vitals and respiratory status.

112. What is the therapeutic blood level of digoxin?

   A. It's 3 mg/mL
   B. It's 2 mg/mL
   C. It's 0.7 ng/mL
   D. It's 6 ng/mL

113. Which is the safe rate needed to rewarm a hypothermia victim with submersion asphyxiation?

    A. 33.8°F/hour
    B. 34.7°F/hour
    C. 35.6°F/hour
    D. 36.5°F/hour

114. What is the primary intervention for a symptomatic myocarditis patient with abnormal heart rhythms on ECG?

    A. IV immunoglobulin
    B. HF medications
    C. Corticosteroids
    D. MRI scan

115. Which is confirmatory for endocarditis diagnosis in a male with h/o drug abuse?

    A. Echocardiogram
    B. CBC
    C. Blood cultures
    D. Chest X-ray

116. What is the priority action in an ICU patient with acute pancreatitis who appears restless and sweating on observation?

    A. Prepare for immediate abdominal USG.
    B. Notify the provider.
    C. Offer pain relief medications.
    D. Assess the vitals and pain levels.

117. Which of these are symptoms of PAH?

    A. Dyspnea
    B. Chest pain
    C. Syncope

D. All of the above

118. Which of these statements is correct concerning pre- and post-renal AKI?

    A. Post-renal AKI is due to urine accumulation.
    B. Pre-renal AKI is due to blockage in the urinary tract.
    C. Post-renal AKI is due to poor perfusion.
    D. Pre-renal AKI is due to bladder injury.

119. Which nursing interventions would *not* improve the cognition of a 79-year-old male with ataxia, memory loss, confusion, and aggression?

    A. Secure and sedate the patient.
    B. Attempt to reorient with the reality.
    C. Ensure environmental safety.
    D. Avoid disputing with the patient.

120. Which patient statement suggests they need more information regarding a new digoxin prescription for HF before discharge?

    A. "I should take a double digoxin dose the next day after I miss it to maintain my levels."
    B. "I must call my primary healthcare provider for fatigue, depression, or squeamishness."
    C. "Even when unwell, I'll take digoxin."
    D. "My primary care provider will specify blood level checks."

121. Which finding rules out acute pulmonary embolism?

    A. PaCO2 49 mmHg
    B. HCO3 25 mmHg
    C. d-dimer 450 micrograms/L
    D. INR 0.8

122. The nurse is caring for a heart failure patient. She finds the client is dyspneic and has crackles on auscultation. Which symptoms can a client with an excess fluid volume show?

    A. Lowered CVP
    B. Flattened neck and hand veins
    C. Weight loss
    D. HTN

123. An inpatient mental health unit client experiences a panic attack while the nurse conducts a group discussion. What is a nurse's most therapeutic action?

    A. Ask other clients to say soothing things to the patient.
    B. Sit with the client and inquire about their feelings.
    C. Take the client to an isolated spot and stay with them.
    D. Move the client to a quiet room and rejoin the group.

124. The nurse is reviewing a client's medical records. Which findings can put the client at risk for hypokalemia?

    A. Burn
    B. Uric acid 10.2 mg/dl
    C. NG suction
    D. H/o Addison's disease

125. A college basketball player is paralyzed from the waist down following a motorbike accident. At the Paralympics, they won gold in wheelchair basketball. What defense mechanism has the athlete used?

    A. Compensation
    B. Anger
    C. Displacement
    D. Acceptance

Answer Key

Q.	1	2	3	4	5	6	7	8	9	10	11	12	13	14
A.	B	D	C	A	B	A	B	D	C	C	C	C	A	C

Q.	15	16	17	18	19	20	21	22	23	24	25	26	27	28
A.	A	A	A	B	A	A	D	A	C	A	B	D	A	C

Q.	29	30	31	32	33	34	35	36	37	38	39	40	41	42
A.	C	A	A	B	B	C	C	C	B	C	C	C	B	A

Q.	43	44	45	46	47	48	49	50	51	52	53	54	55	56
A.	B	A	D	B	D	C	D	B	C	D	A	A	A	B

Q.	57	58	59	60	61	62	63	64	65	66	67	68	69	70
A.	A	D	C	C	B	A	A	A	B	D	A	B	B	A

Q.	71	72	73	74	75	76	77	78	79	80	81	82	83	84
A.	A	A	A	C	A	A	B	D	D	D	B	C	A	D

Q.	85	86	87	88	89	90	91	92	93	94	95	96	97	98
A.	D	D	D	D	C	D	B	A	A	B	B	A	C	D

Q.	99	100	101	102	103	104	105	106	107	108	109	110	111	112
A.	B	D	B	C	C	D	D	D	B	A	C	C	C	D

Q.	113	114	115	116	117	118	119	120	121	122	123	124	125
A.	D	C	A	B	C	B	D	A	A	A	C	D	C

Answer Key and Explanations

1. B. The murmur of aortic stenosis heard at the right second ICS.

2. D. Contraction of pulmonary vessels will allow redistribution of blood flow to unobstructed areas and compensate VQ shunting.

3. C. Symptoms of cardiac tamponade are muffled heart sounds, dilated neck veins, raised CVP, and lowered BP.

4. A. The ECG findings correspond to supraventricular tachycardia.

5. B. Eptifibatide reduces platelet binding, lasting for six hours.

6. A. Common complications following endarterectomy include hematoma, hyper/hypotension, hyperperfusion syndrome, hemorrhage, headache, and stroke. Hematuria is unlikely.

7. B. Vitamin K reverses warfarin action.

8. D. A case of respiratory acidosis. Abnormal pH goes against COPD as a cause.

9. C. Establish an IV line.

10. C. Elder abuse is more likely due to the patient's advanced age and long-term residence in a care institution.

11. C. Check patient information before medication.

12. C. The minimum urine output for this patient should be 468 ml. The minimum urine output for any individual is *0.5 mL/kg/hour*. For a 78 kg patient for 12 hours, it will be 468 mL (78×0.5×12).

13. A. A urine specific gravity 1.030 is not expected in DI.

14.   C. Normal specific gravity is 1.005–1.030.

15.   A. Lowering the frequency raises TV and helps CO2 elimination.

16.   A. Hypernatremia is a risk factor for HHNK.

17.   A. Dementia is a risk for increase in falls.

18.   B. Asking about the last meal is unrelated to the patient's condition, DKA.

19.   A. Patients cannot discontinue atenolol suddenly, precipitating complications.

20.   A. The risk of hypertensive encephalopathy is more in a middle-aged HTN male who has discontinued his antihypertensive medication.

21.   D. Paradoxical breathing is always abnormal in adults, irrespective of yoga practice.

22.   A. Grade III subarachnoid hemorrhage presents with drowsiness, confusion and mild focal neurological deficit.

23.   C. Intracranial hemorrhage is a catastrophic consequence of low platelet levels.

24.   A. Risk for intracranial hemorrhage increases when platelet count is below 20.000 cu/mL.

25.   B. FEV1/FVC 65% (low) indicates COPD.

26.   D. Irregular EEG wave pattern is not a brain death criterion.

27.   A. Balloon inflation compresses plaque/obstruction against the arterial wall, broadening it and improving blood flow.

28.   C. Erythropoietin increases red blood cell counts.

29.   C. A 2/4 twitch corresponds to 90% neuromuscular blockade.

30.   A. tPA is split into 10% of the total dose as a bolus over a minute, followed by 90% over 60 minutes.

31.   A. Fluid resuscitation is a priority in DKA management.

32.   B. Avoid PO challenge when there is a suspicion of bowel obstruction.

33.   B. Report to the doctor to identify and swiftly treat possible retroperitoneal bleeding.

34.   C. β-selective agonists as inhalers are primary management in acute asthma.

35.   C. The least endotracheal tube cuff pressure to prevent aspiration is 20 cm H2O

36.   C. The subjective nature of pain requires self-reporting as the gold standard and accurate pain measurement criterion.

37.   B. PaO2/FiO2 is the percent of inspired oxygen that the patient receives expressed as a decimal: 82/0.4 (40% O2) or 205.

38.   C. Second-degree AV block, Type I, shows blocked atrial beats.

39.   C. PaO2/FiO2<300 suggests acute respiratory failure.

40.   C. Patients will be placed on strict bed rest orders for several hours following the valve replacement procedure.

41.   B. High FiO2 increases dead space in COPD.

42.   A. Diphenhydramine can worsen prolonged QT interval.

43.   B. Paradoxical breathing means urgent need for mechanical ventilation.

44.   A. The most commonly used vessel for femoral-popliteal bypass is the saphenous vein.

45.   D. Inform the provider if the platelet count is < 50,000 platelets/mcL in

a heparinized patient.

46.   B. Sublingual nitroglycerin is effective within one to five minutes.

47.   D. Inhalation is the most effective route for bronchodilator administration.

48.   C. Only short-acting regular insulin is used to treat DKA

49.   D. Avoid acidic foods like tomatoes.

50.   B. The Berlin definition of ARDS states PaO2/FiO2<100 as severe hypoxia.

51.   C. Respiratory acidosis (PaCO2 65) indicates an acute or chronic respiratory failure in this patient.

52.   D. Stop transfusion immediately.

53.   A. Guillain-Barré syndrome may occur after a viral illness/following immunization.

54.   A. Atrial kick produces 20% of CO.

55.   A. Status epilepticus is a medical emergency requiring immediate professional care.

56.   B. Surgery is the last resort.

57.   A. Sedating the patient will reduce auto-PEEP.

58.   D. Fluid retention is 2200 - 1200 = 1000 ml. One liter of fluid corresponds to 2.2 lb of body weight.

59.   C. Compartment syndrome is pressure build-up from internal bleeding.

60.   C. Streptococcus pneumoniae causes bacterial meningitis.

61.   B. Inform the provider.

62.   A. Blood level>40 µg/mL is phenobarbital toxicity.

63. A. Levothyroxine has a narrow therapeutic index.

64. A. Oxygenation is a priority in managing pulmonary edemA.

65. B. An asthma patient unable to finish a sentence needs ICU monitoring.

66. D. Communicate with the interprofessional team to reduce reperfusion delay.

67. A. MI prognosis is better with early intervention.

68. B. Supplemental oxygenation is needed if the pulse oximetry is < 94% in the room air.

69. B. Adenosine can cause asystole and must be considered.

70. A. Atelectrauma is shearing lung injury due to a ventilator.

71. A. Increased CVP indicates compartment syndrome; others will fall.

72. A. Normal EFis>50%.

73. A. CO is HR × SV, or, 5 L/minute.

74. C. Give supplemental oxygen.

75. A. De-escalation techniques demand active listening and providing comfort.

76. A. The 6MWT is the most common test to assess gait and mobility.

77. B. Withholding diuretic medications would increase fluid overload.

78. D. All of the conditions are valid under Medicaid plan B.

79. D. The immediate management of AFib is resetting and controlling cardiac rhythm.

80.	D. Weight reduction and oxygen via C-PAP/BiPAP

81.	B. Idiopathic rise of pulmonary vascular resistance is classified as PAH.

82.	C. Monitor the aPTT and anti-Xa for clotting time and plasma heparin concentration.

83.	A. Discharge advice must be both verbal and written.

84.	D. Raise the pressure limit to increase TV.

85.	D. Inhaled steroids are appropriate for the long-term management of an elderly, uncontrolled asthma patient.

86.	D. Check physical restraints every 15 minutes up to the first hour.

87.	D. Sunscreen prevents photosensitization in patients on chlorothiazide.

88.	D. WPW is a congenital SVT that may manifest in early adulthood.

89.	C. Facial petechiae, facial cyanosis, and V-shaped throat marks suggest manual strangulation.

90.	D. The patient is probably having unstable angina with MI risk.

91.	B. Diastole comprises 2/3 of a cardiac cycle.

92.	A. A patient must lie flat for six hours after a femoral entry interventional cardiac catheterization.

93.	A. Constant hiccuping may indicate displacement of leads with phrenic nerve irritation.

94.	B. Blurred vision can signify hyperglycemia.

95.	B. MAP is DP + 1/3 (SP-DP) or 90 mm Hg.

96. A. CI = CO/BSA or 3.6 L/min/m2.

97. C. Uncompensated respiratory acidosis is characterized by a pH < 7.35, PaCO2 > 45 mm Hg, and HCO3 between 22–26.

98. D. Benzodiazepines are the most common chemical restraints.

99. B. The patient is at a high risk for pyelonephritis.

100. D. Benzodiazepines are most common chemical restraints.

101. B. The patient is at a high risk for pyelonephritis

102. C. A colonoscopic biopsy helps diagnose IBD.

103. C. Rotate insulin injection sites regularly to prevent hypoglycemiA.

104. D. Lying flat helps to prevent bleeding both internally and externally.

105. D. A positive Homan's sign indicates DVT.

106. D. Minimum MAP needed for tissue perfusion is 60 mm Hg.

107. B. Inform the primary provider.

108. A. Urgent fluid restoration is necessary to stabilize hemodynamics.

109. C. Notify the provider to rule out possible pneumothorax.

110. C. A 75% coronary artery occlusion causes anginal discomfort.

111. C. Assess electrolytes, which can cause several symptoms in the elderly.

112. D. Request an OTC prescription for urgent medications from the doctor.

113. D. Assess vitals and respiratory status to avoid complications post-CABG.

114.   C. The therapeutic blood level of digoxin is 0.5–2.0 ng/mL.

115.   A. Raise the body temperature by 33.8°F/hour (1°C/hr).

116.   B. HF medications comprise the main intervention for myocarditis management.

117.   C. Positive blood cultures are confirmatory for endocarditis diagnosis.

118.   B. Inform the primary provider for definitive actions.

119.   D. All are symptoms of PAH.

120.   A. Blockages in the urinary tract can create a backflow and post-renal failure.

121.   A. Restraining and sedating dementia patients may increase symptoms and prolong disorientation.

122.   A. Do not repeat missed/unknown dose or take double the amount to prevent digoxin toxicity.

123.   C. A d-dimer < 500 mcg/L can rule out acute pulmonary embolism.

124.   D. Hypertension indicates a state of excess fluid volume or fluid overload. Others suggest a volume deficit.

125.   C. The nurse should accompany the client to another room and stay with them.

126.   C. NG suction can cause loss of gastrointestinal fluids and cause hypokalemia.

127.   A. Excelling in an area when another area is unreachable, either in the real world or perceived, is defined as compensation. It can be beneficial or detrimental, depending on the chosen technique.

Chapter Eight: Practice Test 2

1.   Which is an NSTEMI risk factor?

   A. BMI 28
   B. Family history of prostate cancer
   C. Uncontrolled HTN
   D. Alcohol addiction

2.   Which pain type indicates MI?

   A. Pressure-like retrosternal pain
   B. Neck pain
   C. Right arm pain
   D. Stabbing chest pain

3.   Which medication stops complete vessel occlusion in MI?

   A. Morphine
   B. Beta-blockers
   C. Nitrates
   D. Statins

4.   What discharge instructions should MI patients receive for nitrate use in acute chest pain?

   A. Before using nitrate, call 911.
   B. Call 911 after using nitrates.

C. After taking sublingual nitrate, call 911 ten minutes later.

D. Dial 911 if no pain relief occurs with three doses of nitrates.

5. What is the minimum prescribed bed rest for myocarditis?

A. Three days

B. Until ECG is normal

C. Until fever disappears

D. Seven days

6. What is the long-term complication of myocarditis?

A. Arrhythmias

B. Unstable angina

C. Chronic heart failure

D. MI

7. What is a PRN order?

A. Daily Lisinopril 10 mg PO

B. Acetaminophen 500 mg PO every 4–6 hours as needed for pain.

C. Quickly administer four chewable aspirin, establish IV access, and get an electrocardiogram.

D. IV cefazolin immediately before cholecystectomy.

8. Which is not required for a medication order?

A. Patient's name

B. Age/date of birth

C. Date and time

D. Name of the dispensing pharmacist

9. Which conditions can have pulsus paradoxus?

A. Cardiac tamponade

B. Severe acute asthma

C. COPD

D. All of the above

10. Which commonly causes health-care-associated diarrhea in older adults?

    A. Shigella
    B. C. difficile
    C. E. coli
    D. Giardia

11. What would you anticipate preparing for a 94-year-old nursing facility patient who became tachypneic while eating and has an opaque, irregular shape on a chest X-ray?

    A. ET
    B. CT scan
    C. Rigid bronchoscopy
    D. MRI

12. What does T stand for in the TIMES framework for wound assessment?

    A. Tissue type
    B. Type of wound
    C. Trauma nature
    D. Thickness of wound

13. What is the muscular strength of a patient with a stroke on a scale of 0–10 who can move his right arm against gravity but not against resistance?

    A. One
    B. Zero
    C. Five
    D. Three

14. In which heart condition can you expect valvular vegetation?

    A. AFib
    B. WPW syndrome
    C. CHF
    D. Endocarditis

15.   Which is NOT a management protocol for sepsis?

   A. Check labs for electrolytes.
   B. Consult a dietitian.
   C. Ensure DVT prophylaxis.
   D. Ensure visitors encourage the patient.

16.   Which food allergies are associated with latex-related (gloves) allergies?

   A. Banana
   B. Kiwi
   C. Avocado
   D. All of them

17.   What should be the first line of management for a patient in the ER with muscle pain and swelling with tea-colored urine following trauma?

   A. Restore fluids.
   B. Administer analgesics.
   C. Provide a warm compress.
   D. Elevate the lower limbs.

18.   What is the most critical period following cardiac surgery?

   A. First hour
   B. 2 to 72 hours
   C. 48 hours
   D. 72 hours

19.   Which is not a risk factor for pressure ulcers?

   A. Age
   B. Immobility
   C. Cognition
   D. Pregnancy

20. Which is not significant for chronic pain assessment?

    A. Pain characteristics
    B. Previous pain medications
    C. Pain radiation
    D. Patient's pain expectations

21. Which nursing action promotes an accurate diagnosis and care plan?

    A. Assessment
    B. Intervention
    C. Outcome
    D. Evaluation

22. Which pain assessment scale is used to understand pain severity?

    A. Wong-Baker Faces scale
    B. McGill Pain Questionnaire
    C. Brief Pain Inventory
    D. Comfort pain scale

23. Which indicates good tissue perfusion following cardiac surgery?

    A. MAP 50 mm Hg
    B. SP 150 mm Hg
    C. Tachycardia
    D. Urine output 0.5 mL/kg/hr

24. What is the purpose of using the analgesic ladder by WHO?

    A. Logical use of analgesics
    B. Links analgesics with pain intensity
    C. Prevents analgesic misuse
    D. All of these

25.   What is the purpose of using a Biobag?

A. To collect urine
B. To relieve headache
C. To treat complex wounds
D. To treat OSA

26.   Which PaO2/FiO2 value indicates moderate ARDS in a pneumonia patient?

A. PaO2/FiO2 < 340 mm Hg
B. PaO2/FiO2 < 280 mm Hg
C. PaO2/FiO2 < 200 mm Hg
D. PaO2/FiO2 < 300 mm Hg

27.   Which is an incorrect abbreviation for drug dispensing?

A. PO
B. SC
C. NG
D. IM

28.   Which is not a nursing diagnosis in ARDS?

A. Ineffective breathing impairing gas exchange
B. Effective airway clearance
C. Aspiration
D. Anxiety

29.   What chest tube drainage amount is considered safe within two to 72 hours following cardiac surgery?

A. Up to 25 ml/hr
B. Up to 50 mL/hr
C. No drainage
D. Up to 70 mL/hr

30. Which patient order for a 72-year-old, 91 kg patient intubated due to progressive ARDS with decreased SaO2 and raised PaCO2 should you question?

     A. Raise PEEP to 12 cmH2O.
     B. Support FiO2 at 100%.
     C. Raise the mechanical tidal volume to 15 mL/kg
     D. Start prone positioning for 16 hours.

31. Which diagnosis applies to a 25-year-old patient with abdominal gunshot wounds, dyspnea, and chest pain? He has tracheal deviation and absent right-side breath sounds.

     A. Subcutaneous emphysema
     B. Pneumopericardium
     C. Tension pneumothorax
     D. Intra-abdominal hemorrhage

32. What diagnostic procedure is definitive for myocarditis?

     A. Transesophageal ultrasound
     B. Transmural catheterization
     C. Chest X-ray
     D. Endomyocardial biopsy

33. Which patient history is significant in asthma?

     A. Age
     B. Atopy
     C. Exercise
     D. Heat intolerance

34. In which situation should you seek assistance in acute asthma management?

     A. SPO2 95%
     B. Rales on auscultation
     C. Silent chest on auscultation

D. RR 18/minute

35. Which heart condition needs antibiotic prophylaxis for surgical procedures?

    A. Arrhythmias
    B. MI
    C. Rheumatic valve disease
    D. Autoimmune heart disease

36. Which is critical to long-term asthma management?

    A. Quit smoking
    B. Exercise more often
    C. Eat healthy
    D. Comply with medications

37. Which is the most significant nursing diagnosis of COPD?

    A. Lack of self-care
    B. Impaired gas exchange
    C. Ineffective breathing pattern
    D. Activity intolerance

38. How many times must you check before administering medications per the rights of medication administration?

    A. Three
    B. Four
    C. Two
    D. One

39. Which intervention is appropriate to address activity tolerance in COPD?

    A. Monitor vitals.
    B. Pace activities with rest.
    C. Administer bronchodilators.

D. Train breathing exercises.

40. Which is not a nursing priority in cardiac cath procedures?

    A. Improving tissue perfusion
    B. Caring for physical health only
    C. Maintaining asepsis
    D. Caring for physical and emotional needs

41. What is the likely diagnosis of an elderly female with hypothyroid and obesity and complaining of daytime sluggishness?

    A. Aggravation of hypothyroid state
    B. OSA
    C. Depression
    D. Electrolyte imbalance

42. What does cardiogenic shock indicate?

    A. Right-sided HF
    B. Left and right-sided HF
    C. Left-sided HF
    D. None of these

43. Which action should you take first if a client is suspected of having avian influenza?

    A. Give the first dose of oseltamivir.
    B. Administer IV fluids.
    C. Administer oxygen using a nonrebreather mask.
    D. Collect blood and sputum specimens.

44. What is the best cleansing solution for skeletal pin site care?

    A. Normal saline
    B. Chlorhexidine 2 mg/mL
    C. Betadine 10%

D. Alcohol 70%

45.   Which substance use can cause dilated CM?

    A. Cocaine
    B. Mescaline
    C. LSD
    D. Heroin

46.   What is narrowed pulse pressure (PP)?

    A. PP < 30 mm Hg
    B. PP < 40 mm Hg
    C. PP < 38 mm Hg
    D. PP < 45 mm Hg

47.   What is the first step while administering prophylactic antibiotics?

    A. Assess the patient's allergy history.
    B. Practice strict hand washing.
    C. Monitor for signs of extravasation.
    D. Ensure on-time administration.

48.   Which dressing is unsuitable for highly exudative wounds?

    A. Transparent film
    B. Alginate
    C. Hydrofiber
    D. Super absorbent polymers (SAPs)

49.   Which is not a non-critical item?

    A. Ice therapy packs
    B. Blood pressure cuffs
    C. Stethoscope
    D. Oral thermometer

50.   Which agent is used for surgical hand antisepsis in the US?

       A. Soap and water
       B. Alcohol-based rub
       C. Povidone iodine
       D. Chlorhexidine

51.   What complication should you monitor for a patient with pulmonary embolism on anticoagulant therapy?

       A. Elevated liver enzymes
       B. Bleeding
       C. Hyperglycemia
       D. Bradycardia

52.   Which sign should alert you to possible endocarditis in a patient with IV substance use?

       A. Janeway lesions
       B. Cyanosis
       C. Tophi
       D. Jaundice

53.   What is your priority action if a patient with PAH has ankle swelling and dyspnea?

       A. Give diuretics.
       B. Prepare for a pulmonary arteriogram.
       C. Assess oxygen saturation.
       D. Request a prescription for anticoagulants.

54.   Which education regarding the use of anticoagulants is vital for a patient with idiopathic PAH on discharge?

       A. Discontinue medication if asymptomatic.
       B. Avoid activities that increase bleeding possibilities.
       C. Use pain relievers.

D. Restrict green leafy veggies.

55.   What type of respiratory failure may occur in a patient with COPD with dyspnea, cyanosis, tachycardia, and SpO2 85%?

A. Obstructive
B. Chronic
C. Hypoxemic
D. Hypercapnic

56.   What is the appropriate initial intervention for a chronic bronchitis patient with increasing confusion, dyspnea, dehydration, fever, and crackles on chest auscultation?

A. Obtain blood cultures.
B. Obtain chest X-ray.
C. Administer antidepressants.
D. Assess and initiate oxygenation.

57.   How much capillary refill time indicates adequate tissue perfusion?

A. Refill time < 5 secs
B. Refill time > 5 secs
C. Refill time < 3 secs
D. Refill time < 6 secs

58.   What is the primary nursing diagnosis for cardiomyopathy?

A. Mental changes
B. Unstable BP
C. Activity intolerance
D. Impaired gas exchange

59.   What advice would you give to manage sugar levels and diabetes while fasting?

A. Avoid all diabetic medications.

B. Avoid fasting.

C. Take the usual insulin dose.

D. Check blood glucose more often.

60. What is the most common cause of pulmonary embolism?

A. DVT

B. SVT

C. PAH

D. CHF

61. Which is not recommended in a CAUTI bundle?

A. Place the drainage bag below the level of the patient's bladder.

B. Insert catheters if patients have urinary incontinence.

C. Obtain routine urine samples from the sampling port.

D. Use clean gloves to insert a Foley catheter.

62. What is a risk factor for a young patient with suspected myocarditis and having dyspnea and chest pain?

A. Gender

B. Age

C. Exposure to infection

D. Previous heart condition

63. Which diagnosis can help assess the pericardial fluid amount in a patient who has developed pericardial effusion two days after cardiac surgery?

A. Cardiac catheterization

B. ECG

C. Echocardiogram

D. Chest X-ray

64. Which is a controlled substance regarding drug administration?

A. Prednisolone

B. Insulin
C. Tylenol
D. Heparin

65.   Which is the most appropriate action for a patient with AAA who is complaining of acute pain and has absent pedal pulses?

A. Assess BP in both arms and alert the physician.
B. Give analgesics and a warm compress.
C. Advise rest.
D. Elevate the foot end of the bed.

66.   Which nursing intervention is appropriate if a patient expresses fear about their scheduled cardiac catheterization?

A. Detail procedural complications
B. Encourage the patient and ask questions
C. Give a sedative
D. Avoid discussion

67.   What is Dressler syndrome?

A. Idiopathic pericarditis
B. Pericarditis following heart attack
C. Infective pericarditis
D. Drug-induced pericarditis

68.   Which is a predictive diagnostic marker for rheumatoid arthritis (RA)?

A. Rheumatoid factor
B. C-reactive protein
C. ESR
D. Anti-CCP (Anti-cyclic citrullinated peptide)

69.   What should the patient's position be to assess their lower limb strength?

A. Lying

B. Sitting

C. Standing

D. Reclining

70. Which finding is consistent with muscle inflammation?

A. Warmth on palpation

B. Spinal deformity

C. Active ROM

D. Foot drop

71. Which antibiotic can cause nephrotoxicity?

A. Aminoglycosides

B. Penicillin

C. Sulphonamides

D. Erythromycin

72. Which drug administration route has the slowest absorption?

A. IM

B. IV

C. Subcutaneous

D. Inhalation

73. Which vein is used for cardiac cath?

A. Iliac vein

B. Femoral vein

C. Saphenous vein

D. Renal vein

74. What is the risk of oxygen therapy?

A. Breathing suppression

B. Inflammation

C. Dehydration

D. None of these

75.   Which order would you question regarding using a Foley catheter?

   A. Use a urinary catheter for urethral trauma.
   B. Ensure dependent loops or kinks are absent.
   C. Wash your hands before handling the drainage bag.
   D. Clean around the catheter with chlorhexidine wipes.

76.   What should be the primary concern before oxygenation?

   A. Saving the patient
   B. Overall safety
   C. Delivery mode
   D. Cost

77.   Which of these statements for sedation by non-anesthesia providers is FALSE?

   A. Non-anesthesia providers can offer sedation to patients with mild systemic disease (PS II) only.
   B. They can sedate patients with severe systemic disease (PS III).
   C. They can sedate healthy individuals (PS I).
   D. Non-anesthesia providers cannot offer sedatives.

78.   What is the functional ability level of a client who needs an assistive device?

   A. Level 1
   B. Level 2
   C. Level 4
   D. Level 3

79.   What is the normal PR interval?

   A. PR ≤ 0.32 secs
   B. PR ≥ 0.35 secs
   C. PR ≤ 0.11 secs

D. PR ≤ 0.22 secs

80. Which adapter should you use in a venturi mask to deliver O2 at 40% FiO2?

   A. Blue
   B. Red
   C. Orange
   D. White

81. Which condition is most likely to present with left-sided diminished breath sounds in a hypertensive smoker presenting with dyspnea and chest pain?

   A. AAA dissection
   B. Pulmonary embolism
   C. Pleural effusion
   D. MI

82. Which patient statement implies their understanding of influenza treatment with an antiviral drug?

   A. I will take the prescription as directed.
   B. I will refrain from infecting others with these medications.
   C. I will stop the drug when I feel well.
   D. I will resume my usual activities.

83. What should you do if a prostate cancer patient wants to know about his diagnosis?

   A. Tell him lies to protect him.
   B. Tell him the truth about his condition.
   C. Ask the provider to communicate.
   D. Ask the family to communicate.

84. Which is not a low-flow O2 delivery system?

    A. Face mask
    B. NRB
    C. Venturi mask
    D. Nasal cannula

85. Which is a likely diagnosis in a smoker with uncontrolled diabetes presenting with loss of hair and sensation on their toes?

    A. Peripheral vascular disease
    B. Diabetic foot
    C. Gangrene
    D. Atherosclerosis

86. Which is a likely diagnosis in a smoker with leg pain and cool skin becoming pale with foot elevation?

    A. Chronic venous insufficiency
    B. May-Thurner syndrome
    C. Peripheral artery disease
    D. DVT

87. Which is a priority diagnostic test in Coronavirus ARDS associated with 102°F temperature, cough, and dyspnea?

    A. ABG analysis
    B. Coronavirus antibody test
    C. Chest X-ray
    D. Viral panel

88. What is the acute management of pulmonary edema if the patient develops blood-stained frothy sputum and orthopnea?

    A. Chest X-ray
    B. HOB elevation
    C. Patient isolation

D. Sedatives

89. What is the primary nursing diagnostic concern for AAA?

   A. Hemorrhage leading to volume deficit
   B. Increased CO
   C. Pain
   D. Insufficient knowledge

90. Who is the highest priority for influenza vaccination?

   A. A 50-year-old man with a hernia
   B. A 36-year-old woman
   C. A 55-year-old man caring for a spouse with cancer
   D. A 60-year-old man with osteoarthritis

91. Which is not a component of moral agency?

   A. Inability to take moral actions
   B. Recognizing ethical concerns
   C. Making moral choice
   D. Inability to take sides in decision-making

92. Which action follows after administering aspirin, nitrates, and heparin to a patient with unstable angina?

   A. CABG preparation
   B. A stat dose of clopidogrel
   C. Oxygen
   D. Monitor complications

93. Which ECG leads show upright T waves?

   A. V2-V6
   B. aVR
   C. aVL
   D. V1-V3

94.   What should you immediately do if a patient with CHF has worsening dyspnea, crackles on chest auscultation, and distended neck veins?

  A. Administer oxygen via nasal cannula.
  B. Administer diuretics.
  C. Start CPAP.
  D. Assess signs of fluid overload.

95.   How would you calculate the atrial rates in ECG?

  A. Number of P waves in 10 seconds.
  B. Number of P waves in 6 secs multiplied by 10.
  C. Number of P waves in 10 secs multiplied by 10.
  D. Number of QRS complexes in 6 seconds multiplied by 10

96.   Which is appropriate preparation for a left-heart cardiac cath in a patient with CAD and on warfarin?

  A. Continue warfarin.
  B. Switch to heparin.
  C. Increase the warfarin dose the night before.
  D. Hold warfarin 48 hrs before surgery.

97.   Which is a sign of inadequate oxygenation and possible oxygen requirement?

  A. Accessory muscle use
  B. Ataxia
  C. Tremors
  D. Sweating

98.   What interface would you choose in a severely hypoxic but ventilating smoke inhalation poisoning patient requiring O2@8L/minute?

  A. Nasal cannula
  B. NRB mask
  C. Face mask

D. Venturi mask

99. Which is not a component of Beck's traid for blunt chest trauma?

   A. Distended neck veins.
   B. Raised temperature.
   C. Muffled heart sounds.
   D. Low BP

100. What should you consider before an extracorporeal membrane oxygenation (ECMO) for managing unresponsive cardiogenic shock?

   A. H/o cardiac tamponade
   B. Cardiac inotropic medication response
   C. Inadequacy of oxygenation
   D. Organ dysfunction

101. What principle guides oxygen therapy?

   A. Administer in all ICU patients.
   B. Use the maximum amount to improve SpO2.
   C. Use the lowest effective dose.
   D. Use a face mask for best results.

102. Which is not a hypoxia sign?

   A. Restlessness
   B. Tachycardia
   C. Confusion
   D. Warm skin

103. How long should a patient sit upright after oral medications?

   A. Ten minutes
   B. Thirty minutes
   C. One hour
   D. Fifteen minutes

104. Which treatment protocol should you anticipate for a patient with increasing AAA?

    A. Resection of aneurysm
    B. Conservative management
    C. Resection and bypass grafting
    D. CABG

105. What should be your priority information to a patient's family about a scheduled cardiac cath if the patient is a known substance user?

    A. Emotional support
    B. Pre- and post-procedural pain management
    C. Procedural risks and benefits
    D. Dietary restrictions

106. What should you assess for an agitated patient in the ER who has dilated pupils, elevated body temperature, and hallucinations?

    A. Assess alcohol intoxication.
    B. Ask about h/o diabetes medications.
    C. Assess vitals.
    D. Auscultate chest for lung infections.

107. Which action is appropriate if a patient with heart failure is sitting on the edge of a bed, sweating excessively, and looking pale?

    A. Arrange an ECG.
    B. Administer nitrates.
    C. Assess vitals and oxygen saturation.
    D. Start oxygenation.

108. What is the diagnosis if a 12-lead ECG shows an atrial rate of 500 beats/ minute, irregular ventricular rates, and F waves?

    A. Atrial flutter
    B. AFib

  C. Atrial tachycardia

  D. 1st degree AV block

109. Which is not an effective fall prevention strategy?

  A. Avoid exercising

  B. Get a vision test done.

  C. Use proper footwear.

  D. Set short-term goals to overcome fears.

110. What is a priority action in a post-op patient with CKD who develops oliguria and raised creatinine?

  A. Administer prescribed diuretics.

  B. Encourage oral fluids.

  C. Assess dehydration signs.

  D. Monitor urine output.

111. Which of these can tall, peaked T waves on an ECG indicate?

  A. Hypocalcemia

  B. NSTEMI

  C. Hyperkalemia

  D. Hyponatremia

112. What is the wound stage if a patient has a penetrating leg wound involving the muscles?

  A. Stage 0

  B. Stage II

  C. Stage I

  D. Stage IV

113. Who should primarily receive training to prevent CLABSI in the ICU?

  A. Bedside nurses

  B. Physicians

C. Cardiologists

D. Internists

114. Which tool helps assess the risks of pressure sores in hospitalized patients?

A. Braden scale

B. Apgar score

C. Clarke's test

D. Bishop's score

115. Which action reflects the best level of caring practice for a patient with CHF with dyspnea and pedal edema?

A. Team collaboration

B. Frequent vitals assessment

C. Medication administration

D. Patient education

116. Which is associated with a heart murmur due to acute valvular regurgitation?

A. S1

B. S3

C. S4

D. S2

117. What should you do when a patient with acute respiratory distress (38 RR) shows accessory muscle use and audible wheezing?

A. Start high-flow nasal cannula oxygen.

B. Prepare for endotracheal intubation.

C. Give oxygen through a non-rebreather mask.

D. Give a beta-blocker.

118. What should you do if a postoperative patient with diabetes has hypogly-cemia signs?

    A. Check glucose levels
    B. Encourage them to eat a meal
    C. Give IV dextrose
    D. Administer insulin

119. Which lead is best to monitor an RBBB?

    A. Lead I
    B. Lead V1
    C. lead V6
    D. Lead II

120. What is your appropriate action if a patient expresses discomfort with a recommended surgical procedure?

    A. Inform the provider.
    B. Assure the procedure has low risks.
    C. Arrange a discussion between the patient and the provider.
    D. Encourage the patient to trust the recommendation.

121. What is the most significant step in managing pressure sores?

    A. Handwashing
    B. Patient repositioning
    C. Antiseptic solutions
    D. Aggressive debridement

122. What should be your action for managing pain in a cancer patient if the patient's family asks for pain medication discontinuation?

    A. Give it without informing the family.
    B. Follow the family's wish.
    C. Consult the primary physician.
    D. Educate the family on pain medication necessity.

123. What is the best practice for disinfecting hands soiled with blood?

    A. Alcohol rub for 15 seconds.
    B. Soap under running water for 15 seconds.
    C. Soap and apply friction under running water for 15 seconds.
    D. Soap, lather, and apply friction under running water for 15 seconds.

124. What is the appropriate action for a patient with MI suddenly reporting dizziness during cardiac cath and 82/50 BP and 120 HR?

    A. Begin CPR.
    B. Assess for bleeding.
    C. Give oxygen.
    D. Check blood sugar level.

125. What is the initial advice if a patient with CHF reports a 2.5 kg weight gain in a week?

    A. Assess fluid retention.
    B. Reduce sodium intake.
    C. Increase diuretics.
    D. Notify the cardiologist.

Answer Key

Q.	1	2	3	4	5	6	7	8	9	10	11	12	13	14
A.	C	A	C	D	B	C	C	D	D	B	C	A	D	D

Q.	15	16	17	18	19	20	21	22	23	24	25	26	27	28
A.	D	D	A	B	D	B	A	A	D	D	C	C	B	B

Q.	29	30	31	32	33	34	35	36	37	38	39	40	41	42
A.	D	C	C	D	B	C	C	D	B	A	B	B	B	C

Q.	43	44	45	46	47	48	49	50	51	52	53	54	55	56
A.	C	B	A	A	A	A	D	B	B	A	C	B	C	D

Q.	57	58	59	60	61	62	63	64	65	66	67	68	69	70
A.	C	C	D	A	B	C	C	C	A	B	B	D	B	A

Q.	71	72	73	74	75	76	77	78	79	80	81	82	83	84
A.	A	D	B	A	A	B	D	A	C	B	C	A	B	C

Q.	85	86	87	88	89	90	91	92	93	94	95	96	97	98
A.	B	C	B	B	A	C	A	D	A	D	B	A	A	B

Q.	99	100	101	102	103	104	105	106	107	108	109	110	111	112
A.	B	D	C	D	B	C	C	A	C	B	A	D	C	D

Q.	113	114	115	116	117	118	119	120	121	122	123	124	125
A.	A	A	A	C	C	C	B	C	B	C	D	C	A

Answer Key and Explanations

1.   C. Uncontrolled HTN is a NSTEMI risk factor.

2.   A. Pain of MI is pressure-like, retrosternal, and radiates along the left arm.

3.   C. Nitrates stop complete vessel occlusion in MI.

4.   D. Dial 911 if there is no pain relief with three doses of nitrates.

5.   B. Bed rest is prescribed until ECG is normal.

6.   C. Myocarditis patients may fully recover, or develop CHF.

7.   C. A PRN order is a medication prescription that is administered when the patient requests or requires it.

8.   D. A medication order doesn't require a pharmacist's name.

9.   D. All of these conditions can have pulsus paradoxus.

10.   B. C. difficile commonly causes health-care-associated diarrhea in older adults.

11.   C. A bronchoscopy can help remove a possible foreign body.

12.   A. T stands for tissue types in the TIMES framework for wound assessment.

13.   D. Muscular movement against gravity but not against resistance is scored three on a scale of 0-10.

14.   D. Infected valvular vegetations are found in endocarditis.

15.   D. To manage sepsis, limit patient visitors.

16.   D. Latex allergy is commonly associated with allergy to bananas, kiwi, and avocado.

17.   A. The likely diagnosis is rhabdomyolysis, requiring fluid resuscitation.

18.   B. Two to 72 hours following cardiac surgery is the most critical period.

19.   D. All are risk factors except pregnancy.

20.   B. Current pain drugs, including pregabalin, opioid analgesics, and acetaminophen, affect patient health, but past drug history is not necessary to assess chronic pain.

21.   A. Nursing assessment helps develop an accurate diagnosis and care plan.

22.   A. Use a Wong-Baker Faces scale to assess pain severity.

23.   D. A urine output of at least 0.5 mL/kg/hr, strong pulses, and warm extremities indicate adequate tissue perfusion.

24.   D. The analgesic ladder helps administer analgesics logically depending upon pain intensity and preventing analgesic misuse.

25.   C. A Biobag (larva) is a dressing used to treat some complex wounds.

26.   C. $PaO_2/FiO_2 < 200$ mm Hg indicates ARDS.

27.   B. It is recommended to avoid abbreviations for subcutaneous to prevent common errors.

28.   B. ARDS has ineffective airway clearance.

29.   D. Up to 70 mL/hr is considered a safe drainage amount.

30.   C. The tidal volume must not exceed 6 mL/kg.

31.   C. The patient has tension pneumothorax.

32.   D. Biopsy is a definitive diagnosis of myocarditis.

33.   B. History of atopy is significant in asthma.

34.   C. Silent chest on auscultation is impending respiratory failure.

35.   C. Rheumatic valve disease with a risk of endocarditis requires procedural antibiotic prophylaxis.

36.   D. Patient compliance with medication is the most significant criterion for successful management.

37.   B. The most significant nursing diagnosis of COPD is impaired gas exchange

38.   A. Nurses must check thrice before administering medications to patients.

39.   B. Pace activities with rest to address activity tolerance in COPD.

40.   B. Cardiac cath can have poor outcomes if patients are tense and afraid.

41.   B. While all can cause sluggishness, patient information points toward OSA as the cause of daytime sluggishness.

42.   C. Cardiogenic shock indicates severe LHF.

43.   C. Initiate oxygenation using a nonrebreather mask.

44.   B. Chlorhexidine 2 mg/mL is best for skeletal pin site care.

45.   A. Cocaine abuse can cause dilated cardiomyopathy.

46.   A. Narrowed PP is < 30 mm Hg

47.   A. Assess the patient's allergy history.

48.   A. Transparent film dressings are unsuitable for highly exudative wounds.

49.   D. Oral thermometer comes in contact with mucus membrane and is a semi-critical item.

50.   B. The Food and Drug Administration (FDA) recommends the strength and potency of alcohol-based rub used for surgical hand antisepsis in the US.

51.   B. Monitor closely for bleeding when a patient is on anticoagulant therapy.

52.   A. Janeway lesions, Osler's nodes, and clubbing indicate endocarditis.

53.   C. Assess oxygen saturation

54.   B. Avoid activities that increase bleeding possibilities.

55.   C. Hypoxemic failure, necessitating prompt oxygenation.

56.   D. Assess and initiate oxygenation.

57.   C. A capillary refill time < 3 secs indicates adequate tissue perfusion.

58.   C. The main nursing diagnosis for cardiomyopathy is activity intolerance.

59.   D. While fasting, checking blood glucose more often is required in patients with diabetes to prevent hypoglycemia.

60.   A. DVT is the most common cause of pulmonary embolism.

61.   B. Catheters are not TOC for incontinence.

62.   C. Exposure to infection can further compromise the condition.

63.   C. An echocardiogram can help determine the amount of pericardial effusion.

64.   C. Tylenol with codeine is a controlled/scheduled substance.

65. A. Assess BP in both arms and alert the physician.

66. B. Encourage the patient and ask questions to alleviate anxiety and fear that can affect the patient's experience poorly.

67. B. Dressler syndrome is pericarditis following heart attack.

68. D. Anti-CCP is a predictive diagnostic marker for RA.

69. B. Patients should be sitting to assess their lower limb strength

70. A. Palpatory warmth/tenderness can signify muscle/joint inflammation.

71. A. Aminoglycosides can cause nephrotoxicity.

72. D. Of the sites mentioned, inhalation is the slowest route of drug absorption.

73. B. A cardiac catheter is usually passed through the femoral vein.

74. A. High oxygen therapy in COPD can cause breathing suppression.

75. A. A Foley catheter is contraindicated in urethral traumA. Hence, you should question an order that recommends using Foley for urethral trauma.

76. B. Safety first is the motto of O2 delivery.

77. D. Non-anesthesia providers offer sedatives to PS I, PS II, and medically well-managed PS III.

78. A. The client has Level 1 functional ability.

79. C. Normal PR interval is ≤ 0.11 secs.

80. B. Use the red adaptor.

81. C. Consider pleural effusion.

82.   A. I will take the medication strictly as prescribed.

83.   B. Tell him the truth about his condition.

84.   C. Venturi mask is used for high-flow O2 delivery.

85.   B. The condition is diabetic foot ulcer.

86.   C. Pallor suggests peripheral artery disease.

87.   B. Confirmation requires a coronavirus antibody test.

88.   B. Elevate the HOB to 30°.

89.   A. Hemorrhage leading to volume deficit is the primary nursing diagnostic concern for AAA.

90.   C. A 55-year-old man caring for a spouse with cancer.

91.   A. Inability to take actions is not a component of moral agency.

92.   D. Monitor the development of complications.

93.   A. V2-V6 shows upright T waves.

94.   D. Assess signs of fluid overload.

95.   B. Number of P waves in 6 secs multiplied by 10 gives atrial rates.

96.   A. Continue warfarin for a left-heart cath to prevent thromboembolic events.

97.   A. Use of accessory muscles implies respiratory distress.

98.   B. An NRB mask is suitable in this case.

99.   B. Raised temperature is not a part of Beck's triad.

100. D. Consider the extent of organ dysfunction before ECMO.

101. C. Use the lowest effective dose.

102. D. Hypoxia will cause cool, clammy, and mottled skin.

103. B. Patients should maintain an upright posture for thirty minutes after oral medications.

104. C. If an AAA increases in size, consider surgical resection and bypass grafting as TOC.

105. C. Discuss procedural risks and benefits to help make informed decisions.

106. A. Assess alcohol intoxication.

107. C. Assess vitals and oxygen saturation.

108. B. The diagnosis is AFib.

109. A. Patients should do graded exercise.

110. D. Monitor urine output.

111. C. Hyperkalemia can show tall, peaked T waves on ECG.

112. D. It is a stage IV wound.

113. A. Bedside nurses are primarily responsible for managing CLABSIs.

114. A. Braden scale helps assess the risk of developing pressure sores.

115. A. Team collaboration reflects the best level of caring practice in health-care management.

116. C. S4 heart sound is associated with compliance.

117.   C. Give oxygen through a non-rebreather mask.

118.   C. Give oral glucose/IV dextrose.

119.   B. Lead V1 is best to monitor an RBBB.

120.   C. Facilitate a discussion between the patient and the provider.

121.   B. Patient repositioning every two hours is the most significant step in managing pressure sores.

122.   C. Consult the primary provider for guidance.

123.   D. For hands soiled with blood/body fluids, soap, lather, and apply friction under running water for 15 seconds.

124.   C. Give oxygen immediately before other interventions.

125.   A. Assess fluid retention and edema.

Chapter Nine: Practice Test 3

1.   Which statement is appropriate to explain synchronized intermittent mandatory ventilation to the patient's family?

   A. It substitutes the patient's natural breathing pattern.
   B. The patient can breathe between the ventilator rates.
   C. It provides a set volume and pressure with each breath.
   D. It gives continuous positive pressure.

2.   Which doesn't align with CLABSI prevention?

   A. Chlorhexidine for skin preparation.
   B. Appropriate hand hygiene.
   C. Not reminding about line removal.
   D. Full barrier precautions

3.   How can you prevent ventilator-associated pneumonia?

   A. Elevate the HOB.
   B. Give antibiotics.
   C. Mouthwash with clean water.
   D. Change drapes regularly.

4.   Which statement shows the patient's understanding of how to prevent chronic bronchitis exacerbations in the future?

    A. I will only use my dust respirator at my job.
    B. I should save my daily bronchodilator medication for breathing difficulties only.
    C. I should avoid common triggers for my bronchitis.
    D. I will reduce smoking.

5.   What is the most critical nursing error?

    A. Falls prevention
    B. Inadequate prioritization
    C. Preparing medications in a special quiet zone
    D. Hourly rounding

6.   Which is a likely diagnosis in a patient with malaise, severe dyspnea, and a syncopal episode? He has a burning retrosternal sensation that worsens when lying down.

    A. Pleural effusion
    B. Myocarditis
    C. Pericardial tamponade
    D. GERD

7.   Which hemodynamic change occurs in cardiac tamponade?

    A. CO increases
    B. Contractility falls
    C. RR reduction
    D. Stroke volume rises

8.   In which condition is Quincke's sign observed?

    A. Mitral Stenosis
    B. Aortic insufficiency
    C. Endocarditis

D. Pericarditis

9.   What is the action of a beta blocker?

A. Increase diastolic filling time.
B. Increase myocardial oxygen demand.
C. Increase heart rate.
D. Increase afterload.

10.   Which leads directly reflect inferior wall infarction?

A. II, aVF
B. I, aVL
C. V1-V2
D. V5-V6

11.   What is a priority action in a hypertensive and diabetic elderly female presenting in the ER with uncontrolled vomiting, dizziness, and a "flip-flop" sensation in her heart?

A. Ensure the ABCs of emergency protocol.
B. Take baseline vitals.
C. Give O2.
D. Initiate continuous ECG monitoring.

12.   What is a priority nursing action if a 25-year-old female patient complaining of chest pain, agitation, and headache, has 180/120 BP?

A. Monitor BP frequently.
B. Administer antihypertensives.
C. Administer O2.
D. Monitor ECG.

13.   The doctor writes a prescription to infuse 300 mL over 5 hours. How many mL should the nurse run the drip hourly?

A. 50 mL/hr

B. 100 mL/hr

C. 60 mL/hr

D. 90 mL/hr

14.   A patient's ABG shows PaO2 88 mm Hg and PaCO2 38 mm Hg. The corresponding values in mixed venous blood gasses are PvO2 40 mm Hg and PvCO2 46 mm Hg. What do these findings suggest?

A. Cardiac output impairment

B. Hemodynamic alteration

C. Inadequate tissue oxygenation

D. Adequate capillary oxygen-carbon dioxide exchange

15.   A 25-year-old female patient has a diagnosis of occipital lobe damage after an automobile accident. What patient support should the nurse anticipate?

A. Ability to feel hot temperatures

B. Determining smells

C. Interpreting visual images

D. Making meaningful conversation

16.   Which is a crucial assessment in an elderly patient with MI who is suddenly complaining of fatigue, exertional dyspnea, and chest pain?

A. HR

B. Cardiac rhythm

C. SpO2

D. All of the above

17.   Which brain area regulates endocrine and autonomic nervous system (ANS) functions?

A. Temporal lobe

B. Basal ganglia

C. Hypothalamus

D. Reticular activating system (RAS)

18. Which scenario describes proper nursing delegation?

   A. Assigning wound assessment for a postoperative patient with increased pain
   B. Quadriplegic patient bathing
   C. Vital sign check in a chest pain patient
   D. Teaching a patient about a new drug order

19. Which leads are appropriate for viewing an anterior wall infarct?

   A. V4, R
   B. V2, V4
   C. V5, V6
   D. V7, V9

20. A pulse oximetry shows a drop in SpO2 from 95% to 85% over several hours. What is the nurse's priority action?

   A. Check the probe's placement on the finger or earlobe.
   B. Promptly order ABG to confirm with a corresponding SaO2.
   C. Start oxygen by nasal cannula at 2 L/min.
   D. Notify the provider.

21. What is the priority nursing assessment for an elderly hypertensive female with confusion and impaired speech?

   A. Cerebral perfusion
   B. Serum electrolytes
   C. Blood sugar values
   D. Renal status

22. The nurse plans to delegate some patient-related tasks at the nursing facility. Which is not related to successfully overseeing the assigned tasks?

   A. Criticism and negative feedback
   B. Problem resolving skills
   C. Prompt follow-ups

D. Excellent communication and leadership skills

23.   The doctor prescribes to infuse 1500 mL of D5W over 12 hours. The drip factor is 20 gtt/mL. How many drops per minute (gtt/min) will the nurse adjust?

A. 30 gtt/min
B. 42 gtt/min
C. 54 gtt/min
D. 25 gtt/min

24.   In which condition pulse oximetry may not be a reliable indicator of oxygen saturation?

A. Fever
B. Hypovolemic shock
C. Anesthetized patients
D. Oxygen therapy

25.   What is the stage of hypertension in a patient with BP 125/89?

A. Stage 1
B. Prehypertension
C. Stage 2
D. Normal BP

26.   Which is a probable condition for a patient with lower extremity numbness who has weak peripheral pulses and diminished BP on both limbs?

A. Intestinal hemorrhage
B. Cardiogenic shock
C. Peripheral arterial disease
D. Stroke

27.   Which is a likely diagnosis if a 58-year-old patient with dengue has tachycardia and 80/50 BP on day 5 of illness?

    A. Dehydration
    B. Dengue shock
    C. MI
    D. UTI

28.   How long should a patient avoid watering a pacemaker insertion site?

    A. Four days
    B. Three days
    C. Seven days
    D. One day

29.   A 75-year-old patient has a SpO2 of 70%. What other assessment should the nurse consider before anticipating adequate oxygenation in this patient?

    A. The oxygenation status with a stress test
    B. Hyperkalemia
    C. The patient's SpO2 values compared to normal values
    D. Current vital signs compared to previous values

30.   Which activity is essential after removing an arterial sheath?

    A. Advise bed rest.
    B. Give O2.
    C. Watch for bleeding.
    D. Assess vitals.

31.   A patient with severe burns is increasingly apprehensive about painful dressing changes. What would be the most appropriate treatment the nurse may ask the provider to prescribe?

    A. Patients should be allowed to control analgesic administration.
    B. Midazolam with morphine before dressing changes.

C. Morphine in a dose range allowing for more before dressing changes.

D. Buprenorphine is given with morphine.

32.   Which medication will probably be prescribed to lower BP?

A. Beta-blockers
B. Dopamine
C. Beta-agonists
D. Epinephrine

33.   Which assessment is vital as a preventative measure in HTN?

A. Headache
B. Pumping activity of the heart.
C. Activity intolerance
D. Pain

34.   Smoking impairs which respiratory defense mechanism the most?

A. Cough reflex
B. Mucociliary movements
C. Air filtration
D. Reflex bronchospasm

35.   How long should a patient fast before pacemaker insertion?

A. Six hours
B. Overnight
C. Eight hours
D. Ten hours

36.   Which can help maintain the contour of the scarring during the burn injury rehabilitation period?

A. Pressure clothing
B. Sunlight avoidance
C. Splinting the joint in extension

D. Emollient lotions

37. Which lab investigation is essential for venous sheath removal?

    A. Serum electrolytes
    B. INR
    C. Serum albumin
    D. Troponin

38. A 28-year-old female patient refuses wound cleaning and dressing change, stating they won't make any difference. How can the nurse facilitate the patient's healing?

    A. Have the wound tended to.
    B. Offer a snack before the procedure.
    C. Discuss her concerns.
    D. Call the chaplain to convince the patient.

39. What dietary advice must you emphasize for hypertensive patients?

    A. Cut back on salt.
    B. Eat less meat.
    C. Eat colorful foods.
    D. Drink fruit juice.

40. What are the functions of the thalamus?

    A. Processing auditory inputs
    B. Integrating past experiences
    C. Relaying sensory and motor input to and from the cortex
    D. Controlling learned and automatic movements

41. What should you monitor following a pacemaker insertion?

    A. Vitals
    B. Breathing
    C. ECG

D. All of the above

42.   What is the first step to initiating defibrillation?

A. Check the ECG.
B. Switch ON the power.
C. Start CPR
D. Choose the paddles.

43.   The patient asks the nurse about what the blood-brain barrier is. What is the best explanation the nurse can offer?

A. Shields the brain from external trauma
B. Protects the brain from dangerous blood-borne agents
C. Offers flexibility while protecting the spinal cord
D. Forms the outer layer of protective membranes

44.   What should the nurse anticipate to find during the neurologic assessment of the older adult?

A. Low intelligence score
B. Absence of deep tendon reflexes
C. Reduced sensation of temperature
D. Less spontaneous awakening

45.   Which patient information is important before a cardiac cath?

A. Assuring them of the physician's competency
B. Telling them they will be alright
C. Explaining the procedure
D. Letting them drink water before the procedure

46. The ICU nurse answers the phone from a stranger who wants to know how one of her patients is doing. What might be the most appropriate step for the nurse?

    A. Review the patient's medical record to verify that the individual is on the approved list to receive patient information.
    B. Enter the individual's details into the patient's record before providing the necessary information.
    C. No information can be given over the phone.
    D. Reassure the patient is receiving excellent treatment.

47. What must you obtain before a cardioversion procedure for a patient with AFib?

    A. Lab electrolyte values (K and Mg)
    B. INR
    C. Patient informed consent
    D. Informed consent with an immediate family member's contact number

48. A woman had a right breast mastectomy. Post-op, her right arm became severely swollen. What hematologic problem is this due to?

    A. Lymphedema
    B. Right arm immobility
    C. Right-sided wound
    D. Right-sided heart failure

49. What is the main function of a pacemaker?

    A. Maintain HR.
    B. Replace normal cardiac pacing.
    C. Lower BP.
    D. Prevent syncope.

50. A patient becomes angry and refuses to take medications. What is the nurse's best statement?

    A. Trust your doctor to make the right decision for you.
    B. I'll get you an extra dessert if you take your medication.
    C. You will always feel better after your medications.
    D. If you disregard your medication, I'll have it given through a feeding tube.

51. Which BP measurement predicts end-organ failure?

    A. SBP drop of 20 mm Hg
    B. MAP drop of 55 mm Hg
    C. SBP drop > 30 mm Hg
    D. MAP drop < 20 mm Hg

52. Which nutrients are important for red blood cell (RBC) production?

    A. Iron
    B. Vitamin C
    C. Vitamin D
    D. Vitamin B 6

53. What is appropriate advice for an HTN patient complaining of reduced exercise tolerance and weakness?

    A. Reduce weight.
    B. Do a sleep test.
    C. Exercise interspersed with rest.
    D. Manage pain.

54. What should the nurse ask the patient when assessing a patient with anemia?

    A. Recent stomach surgery
    B. Corticosteroid treatment
    C. MI

D. Oral contraceptive use

55. What is the first step before managing hypertensive crisis with vasoactive drugs?

    A. Treat hypovolemia.
    B. Give O2.
    C. Give IV antihypertensives.
    D. Announce code blue.

56. What is the most critical effect of intracranial hypertension?

    A. Infection
    B. Herniation
    C. Sensory loss
    D. Motor loss

57. A patient with a hematologic disorder has a smooth, shiny, red tongue. Which laboratory result is expected?

    A. Neutrophils 55%
    B. WBC count 13,500
    C. Hb 9.5 g/dL
    D. RBC count 6.5×10^6 /μL

58. A patient is on chemotherapy. Which result should the nurse review in the patient's care plan?

    A. WBC count 4000/μL
    B. Platelets 50,000/μL
    C. RBC count 3.8 × 106 /μL
    D. Hematocrit (Hct) 39%

59. Which advice must you give to a patient after pacemaker insertion?

    A. Avoid contact sports for a month.
    B. Take waking radial pulse twice weekly.

C. Wear a MedicAlert bracelet.
D. Remain mostly on bed rest.

60. When teaching the patient with angina about sublingual nitroglycerin tablets, what should the nurse tell the patient?

A. Lie or sit and keep a tablet under the tongue during chest pain.
B. Take the tablet with a large quantity of water.
C. Attend ER if one tablet does not relieve the pain in 15 minutes.
D. Stop the medication if it causes dizziness and headache, and inform the provider.

61. What would the nurse anticipate to find during the physical assessment of a patient with thrombocytopenia?

A. Sternal pain
B. Jaundiced sclera
C. Petechiae and purpura
D. Tender, swollen lymph nodes

62. Which assessment is implied if you're asked to monitor the "hemodynamics" of a patient?

A. Vitals
B. Urine output
C. Capillary refill time
D. All of the above

63. Which recommendations does the nurse implement while instructing a senior citizen with CAD in managing their angina treatment plan?

A. Sit for two to five minutes before standing when leaving the bed.
B. Exercise only twice a week.
C. Lifestyle changes are only for a younger person.
D. Aspirin therapy is contraindicated in older adults.

64. When are catecholamine tests ordered?

    A. To rule our stress
    B. To diagnose tumors
    C. For anaphylaxis
    D. To diagnose Parkinson's

65. Why must unstable angina be recognized and treated promptly in any patient with chest pain?

    A. Severe and disabling pain
    B. ECG changes and dysrhythmias
    C. Complete thrombus can occlude the vessel lumen
    D. Risk of MI

66. What should you reply if a patient asks you why he's having a PCI?

    A. You will be able to run again.
    B. To open blocked coronary arteries.
    C. The doctor knows better.
    D. To cure his MI.

67. The nurse suspects stable angina instead of MI in a patient with chest pain. What is her assumption based on?

    A. The pain is relieved by nitroglycerin.
    B. Lack of radiation to the neck, back, or arms.
    C. A sensation of tightness is present.
    D. Pain started after physical exertion.

68. What is normal CVP?

    A. CVP: 15 mm Hg
    B. CVP: 6 mm Hg
    C. CVP: 12 mm Hg
    D. CVP: 9 mm Hg

69.   A 45-year-old female patient has a sudden drop in heart rate while being suctioned through an endotracheal tube. What should the nurse do?

   A. Cease suctioning; administer 100% oxygen.
   B. Suction and administer 100% oxygen.
   C. Turn the head to the right side.
   D. Push saline through the tube to remove the mucus plug.

70.   What is the initiating dose of dopamine infusion?

   A. 5 mcg/kg/min
   B. 2 mcg/kg/min
   C. 8 mcg/kg/min
   D. 10 mcg/kg/min

71.   Which is the first-line drug to treat shock due to unknown causes?

   A. Dobutamine
   B. Epinephrine
   C. Dopamine
   D. Adrenaline

72.   Which hypertensive medication requires the patient to take enough potassium in their diet?

   A. Calcium-channel blocker
   B. Spironolactone
   C. Labetalol
   D. Hydrochlorothiazide

73.   What can be a crucial intervention to promote healing in a patient with viral hepatitis?

   A. Ensuring adequate nutritional intake
   B. Enforcing absolute bed rest during the icteric phase
   C. Providing pain alleviation excluding liver-metabolized drugs
   D. Choosing gentle activities suitable for extreme fatigue

74. How much insulin must you mix to make an infusion?

    A. 280 IU
    B. 200 IU
    C. 250 IU
    D. 180 IU

75. What is the correct technique for BP measurements?

    A. Take the BP in both arms.
    B. Position the patient supine.
    C. Tie the cuff loosely around the upper arm.
    D. Take at least two readings one minute apart.

76. Which laboratory result corresponds to cirrhosis?

    A. Serum albumin: 7.4 g/dL
    B. Total bilirubin: 3.5 mg/dL
    C. Serum cholesterol: 270 mg/dL
    D. Aspartate aminotransferase (AST): 6.0 U/L

77. The doctor prescribes 0.1 grams of medication by mouth daily. The pharmacy dispenses 100 mg per tablet. How many tablets will the nurse give per dose?

    A. One
    B. Two
    C. One-fourth
    D. One half

78. A patient with cirrhosis unresponsive to other esophageal varices treatments receives a portacaval shunt. How can the nurse explain its benefit to the patient?

    A. Survival rate improvement
    B. Nutritional improvement
    C. Serum ammonia level reduction
    D. Renal perfusion improvement

79.   What task can the nurse delegate to the unlicensed assistive personnel (UAP)?

      A. Dispense antihypertensive medications to stable patients.
      B. Measure orthostatic blood pressure (BP) readings for older patients.
      C. Check the BP of a patient on IV enalapril.
      D. Teach home BP monitoring.

80.   What is the medium for preparing a dobutamine infusion for cardiogenic shock?

      A. Normal saline
      B. D5W
      C. D2.5W
      D. Ringer's Lactate

81.   What should the nurse advise a patient with alcoholic cirrhosis regarding long-term management?

      A. A daily exercise regimen.
      B. Cirrhosis can be reversed with proper rest and nutrition.
      C. Abstinence from alcohol.
      D. Acetaminophen is the only over-the-counter analgesic allowed.

82.   A female patient asks the nurse why she needs surgery for a strangulated femoral hernia. What is the most reasonable explanation the nurse can offer?

      A. It will cure her constipation.
      B. The atypical hernia must return to the abdomen.
      C. The surgery will prevent gut necrosis.
      D. The anomalous congenital umbilical opening must be closed.

83.   Which indicates a patient is having a hypertensive emergency?

      A. Stroke with an elevated BP
      B. A BP of 210/124 mm Hg

C. A sudden rise in BP with neurological findings

D. A significant BP elevation over several days or weeks

84. What information should the nurse teach a patient about colostomy irrigation?

    A. Use 1500 to 2000 mL of warm tap water for irrigation.
    B. Allow 30 to 45 minutes for the infusate to remain inside to expel the feces.
    C. Pass a firm plastic catheter four inches into the stoma opening.
    D. Suspend the irrigation bag on a hook 36 inches above the stoma.

85. A 22-year-old woman with PID expresses her fear that the illness will prevent her from becoming a mother. How should the nurse respond to the patient?

    A. For now, I would forget that. Curing your infection is our primary objective.
    B. It is too early to predict. However, infertility following PID is not frequent.
    C. Shall we have a conversation about its significance for you?
    D. You should worry about other significant PID-related complications like abscesses.

86. Which insulin is used to make an infusion to manage DKA?

    A. Long-acting
    B. Regular
    C. Intermediate-acting
    D. Rapid-acting

87. What is a potential adverse effect of palpating an enlarged thyroid gland?

    A. Carotid artery compression
    B. Cricoid cartilage damage
    C. Disproportionate thyroid hormone release into circulation
    D. Hoarseness due to recurrent laryngeal nerve compression

88.   What may the nurse find when examining a patient eight hours after a colostomy?

A. Hyperactive bowel sounds.
B. A brick-red, swollen stoma oozing blood
C. A purplish, moist, and shiny with mucus stoma
D. A small quantity of stomal liquid fecal drainage

89.   Which drugs are typically used to treat hypertensive crises?

A. Esmolol and captopril
B. Enalaprilat and minoxidil
C. Labetalol and bumetanide
D. Intravenous Fenoldopam and sodium nitroprusside

90.   A woman undergoing a total abdominal hysterectomy at the age of 47 wants to know if she can take estrogen until menopause. How should the nurse answer?

A. It will help avoid more severe symptoms associated with surgically induced menopause.
B. You may not require extra estrogen as you are approaching the normal menopause period.
C. Your ovaries, which will not be removed, will continue to secrete estrogen until your normal menopause.
D. Estrogen replacement therapy has many hazards.

91.   Which solution is used to make an insulin infusion?

A. Normal saline
B. Ringers'
C. D5W
D. D2.5W

92.   A patient with a 10-week pregnancy presents with vaginal bleeding and abdominal cramping. What is the nurse's assumption?

    A. It is normal in early pregnancy.
    B. The patient probably has a spontaneous abortion.
    C. The patient will be prepared for a dilation and curettage (D&C).
    D. Complete bed rest will prevent further bleeding.

93.   Which is an essential nursing intervention for a patient with a small intestinal obstruction with an NG tube?

    A. Provide ice chips to suck PRN.
    B. Give hourly mouth care.
    C. Rinse the tube every six hours.
    D. Supine positioning with the HOB elevated 30 degrees.

94.   The nurse initially titrates the medications when treating a patient with a BP of 222/148 with confusion, nausea, and vomiting. Which goal does this achieve?

    A. Reduce the MAP to 129 mm Hg.
    B. Lower the BP within the normal range in two hours.
    C. Reduce the BP 158/111 mm Hg within two hours.
    D. Decrease BP to 160/100 and 110 mm Hg quickly.

95.   How would you measure the QT interval in ECG?

    A. P-P interval
    B. R-R interval
    C. P-Q interval
    D. Q-T interval

96.   A patient with abdominal pain and irregular vaginal bleeding is admitted as suspected ectopic pregnancy. What is the most appropriate action by the nurse?

    A. Provide analgesics.

    B. Monitor vital signs, pain, and bleeding.

    C. Explain frequent blood sample monitoring.

    D. Offer emotional support.

97. Which nursing practice helps problem-solving with excellent scientific data from patient and practitioner experiences?

    A. Quality improvement (QI)

    B. Systematic investigations

    C. Research

    D. Evidence-based practice (EBP)

98. Which drug can prolong QT interval?

    A. Beta-blockers

    B. Escitalopram

    C. Sotalol

    D. Cephalosporins

99. The doctor prescribes a liquid oral medication for a sore throat. The prescription mentions administering 30 mg orally every 4 hours. The pharmacy dispenses 120 mg/5ml. How many ml will the nurse administer per dose?

    A. 1.25 ml/dose

    B. 0.5 ml/dose

    C. 3 ml/dose

    D. 0.8 ml/dose

100. What treatment does the nursing plan include for a patient with appendicitis developing peritonitis as a complication?

    A. IV fluid replenishment

    B. Peritoneal lavage

    C. Peritoneal dialysis

    D. Additional oral fluid intake

101. Which presentations may alert the nurse specifically to endocrine dysfunction?

    A. Goiter and alopecia
    B. Exophthalmos and tremors
    C. Weight loss, fatigue, and depression
    D. Polyuria, polydipsia, and polyphagia.

102. Which of these describes a complex wound?

    A. More than a month old
    B. Slightly contaminated
    C. Closed wounds
    D. Diabetic foot ulcers

103. Which intervention is not appropriate for caring for a client with disruptive behavior?

    A. Involve clients and families in therapy.
    B. Help the client develop self-esteem and coping abilities.
    C. Allow socializing.
    D. Isolate the client.

104. Which is not a medication for procedural sedation?

    A. Buprenorphine
    B. Midazolam
    C. Fentanyl
    D. Diazepam

105. How long should the nurse instruct a patient with diabetes to fast for accurate results of a fasting blood glucose analysis?

    A. Two hours
    B. Eight hours
    C. Six hours
    D. Twelve hours

106.   Which is the "D" of the delirium risk factor screening?

   A. Diarrhea
   B. Dehydration
   C. Dizziness
   D. Disquiet

107.   Which is not an appropriate intervention for altered mental state management?

   A. Stimulate the patient.
   B. Install safety measures.
   C. Maintain routine.
   D. Limit napping.

108.   Which endocrine problems due to hypothyroidism in older adults can be mistakenly attributed to aging?

   A. Tremors and numbness
   B. Fatigue and mental slowing
   C. Hyperpigmentation and slippery skin
   D. Fluid accumulation and hypertension

109.   Which symptom indicates a possible beta-blocker toxicity in an asthma patient?

   A. Urticaria
   B. Reduced urine output
   C. Tachycardia
   D. Vomiting

110.   What is an essential understanding of palliative care?

   A. There are no perfect words/interventions; be present.
   B. Discourage reminiscing.
   C. Ask the patient to accept their fate.
   D. Remind the family that they shouldn't show their grief to the client.

111. Which assessment findings may the nurse find in a female patient admitted with a new diagnosis of Cushing syndrome with elevated serum and urine cortisol levels?

    A. Hair loss and moon face
    B. Reduced weight and hirsutism
    C. Decreased muscle mass
    D. High BP and blood glucose

112. Which component of a mental status assessment of the older adult is critical?

    A. Federal health program eligibility
    B. Prospect for independent living
    C. Service and placement requirements
    D. Categorization as a frail individual

113. What is crucial in older adult rehabilitation to prevent loss of function from inactivity and immobility?

    A. Assistive device utilization
    B. Healthy diet instruction to prevent muscle mass loss
    C. Active and passive range-of-motion (ROM) exercises
    D. Risk appraisals and assessments concerning immobility

114. A patient with type 1 diabetes checks his long-term glycemic control. Which test should he use?

    A. Glycosylated hemoglobin (A1C)
    B. Water deprivation test
    C. Fasting blood glucose
    D. Oral glucose tolerance test

115. A prescription says to give a patient with constipation 4 tsp of laxative. How much is this in mL?

    A. 5 ml

B. 10 ml
C. 20 ml
D. 15 ml

116. The nurse is caring for a patient with a severe flare-up of inflammatory bowel disease. The physician has prescribed an enema with betamethasone. Which of these is the commonly used type of enema to give this medication?

A. Return-flow enema
B. Carminative enema
C. Cleansing enema
D. Retention enema

117. You are caring for a severe trauma patient with a Foley catheter. During your shift, the patient produced 150 cc of urine. In the past 24 hours, urine volume was 350 cc. Which diagnosis would you anticipate?

A. Anuria
B. Polyuria
C. Dysuria
D. Oliguria

118. A middle-aged female with Meniere's disease has a severe attack of the condition following an admission for another illness. Which assistive devices would be *least* helpful to implement into the nursing care plan?

A. A shower chair
B. A walker
C. A sound amplifier
D. A utensil cuff

119. A patient receives a prescription for pen-filled insulin. What should the nurse advise regarding its storage?

A. Keep the pen in the fridge.
B. Do not shake the pen before the administration.

C. Keep the pen in a dry and dark place at room temperature.
D. Always apply the injection at the same site.

120. Which of the following is the leading cause of end-stage renal disease (ESRD)?

    A. Pyelonephritis
    B. Diabetic nephropathy
    C. Diabetes insipidus
    D. Diabetes mellitus

121. What does a low-pitched rumbling murmur signify on auscultation?

    A. Atrial septal defect
    B. Mitral insufficiency
    C. Mitral stenosis
    D. Heart failure

122. What is the complication of administering a hypertonic IV glucose solution to a hypoglycemic patient?

    A. Thrombophlebitis
    B. Hypokalemia
    C. Hyperglycemia
    D. Vascular collapse

123. A probiotic prescription mentions 25,000 mcg of lactobacillus. How much does this mean in mg?

    A. 250 mg
    B. 25 mg
    C. 250,000mg
    D. 2.5 mg

124. Bedside dysphagia assessment involves all of these EXCEPT?

    A. Rely on a gag reaction to decide feeding time.

B. Check for coughing or choking when eating and drinking.

C. Check pharyngeal reflex.

D. Assess face muscle strength.

125.   Which is not indicated in the enteral feeding protocol?

A. Check feeding tube integrity at the end of your shift.

B. Assess HR for refeeding syndrome in chronic malnutrition.

C. Flush the tube with a specified quantity of water.

D. Monitor bowel sounds.

Answer Key

Q.	1	2	3	4	5	6	7	8	9	10	11	12	13	14
A.	B	C	A	C	B	B	B	B	A	A	A	A	C	D

Q.	15	16	17	18	19	20	21	22	23	24	25	26	27	28
A.	C	D	C	B	B	A	A	A	B	B	B	C	B	B

Q.	29	30	31	32	33	34	35	36	37	38	39	40	41	42
A.	D	C	B	A	B	B	C	A	B	C	A	C	D	A

Q.	43	44	45	46	47	48	49	50	51	52	53	54	55	56
A.	B	C	C	A	D	A	A	C	C	A	C	A	A	B

Q.	57	58	59	60	61	62	63	64	65	66	67	68	69	70
A.	C	C	C	A	C	D	A	B	C	B	A	B	B	A

Q.	71	72	73	74	75	76	77	78	79	80	81	82	83	84
A.	C	D	A	C	D	B	A	D	B	B	C	C	C	B

Q.	85	86	87	88	89	90	91	92	93	94	95	96	97	98
A.	C	B	C	B	D	C	A	B	B	A	B	B	D	C

Q.	99	100	101	102	103	104	105	106	107	108	109	110	111	112
A.	A	A	D	D	D	A	B	B	A	B	C	A	D	B

Q.	113	114	115	116	117	118	119	120	121	122	123	124	125
A.	C	A	C	D	D	D	C	B	C	A	B	A	A

Answer Key and Explanations

1. B. The patient can breathe between the ventilator rates while the ventilator gives additional set rates.

2. C. Ask daily if the line can be removed.

3. A. Elevate the HOB.

4. C. I should avoid common triggers for my bronchitis.

5. B. Inadequate prioritization can lead to fatal consequences.

6. B. Burning retrosternal pain that worsens when supine is a cardinal symptom of myocarditis.

7. B. Cardiac contractility falls in cardiac tamponade.

8. B. Quincke's sign of aortic insufficiency is a visible pulsation in the nail bed when pressing down on the finger top.

9. A. Beta blockers raise diastolic filling time.

10. A. II, and aVF represent the inferior heart.

11. A. The patient probably has dysrhythmias. While all are essential, establishing the ABCs of emergency protocol is a priority action.

12. A. Frequent blood pressure monitoring, calming the patient, and notifying the provider are priority nursing actions.

13. C. The nurse should adjust the drip @ 60 mL/hr (300/5).

14. D. The values reflect adequate capillary oxygen-carbon dioxide exchange. Venous blood gas values show O2 uptake from arterial blood and CO2 release from the cells into the blooD. It will have lower PaO2 and raised PaCO2 than arterial blood.

15.   C. The occipital lobes help with visual perception. The patient may have trouble identifying colors, hallucinations, vision loss, or total blindness.

16.   D. The patient is probably having heart failure and requires monitoring of cardiopulmonary response to activity.

17.   C. Hypothalamus regulates endocrine and ANS functions.

18.   B. Nursing assistants help nurses with everyday tasks on stabilized patients.

19.   B. V2, and V4 represent the anterior wall of the heart.

20.   A. Pulse oximetry gives inaccurate readings if the probe is loose. Before taking other measures, the nurse should check the probe position.

21.   A. Assess the Glasgow coma scale for confusion; look for signs of reduced brain perfusion.

22.   A. A successful supervisor must not use criticism and negative feedback to manage staff.

23.   B. The nurse will administer 125 mL/hr or 2.08 mL/minute. If 20 drops make one mL, the nurse should run the drip @ 41 gtt/min.

24.   B. The hypovolemic shock causes poor peripheral perfusion. Pulse oximetry would be inaccurate in this situation.

25.   B. The patient is in the prehypertension stage.

26.   C. The patient has peripheral arterial disease (PAD).

27.   B. The condition is likely dengue shock syndrome.

28.   B. Patients should avoid watering a pacemaker insertion site for three days.

29.   D. Vital signs will change with decreased oxygenation compared to the patient's previous results. Comparing SpO2 with normal values may not be helpful in older patients or patients with respiratory disease. The stress test is not applicable in the current scenario.

30.   C. The main aim is monitoring and preventing bleeding.

31.   B. Midazolam causes short-term memory loss, and if administered before a dressing change, the patient will not recall the procedure. Buprenorphine antagonizes morphine action. Others do not help relieve discomfort during dressing.

32.   A. Beta-blockers (negative inotropes) reduce cardiac workload and BP.

33.   B. Nurses must determine the contributory factors for cardiac function restrictions (rhythm, pace, BP, and activities that reduce cardiac burden).

34.   B. Smoking impairs the mucociliary clearance system.

35.   C. An eight-hour fasting is required for pacemaker insertion.

36.   A. Pressure garments can keep the scars at the original burn injury area level.

37.   B. Assessing the patient's bleeding and coagulation profile is essential before venous/arterial sheath removal.

38.   C. It is natural for burn victims to lose confidence in the healing process. The nurse must empathically communicate with the patient about their concerns.

39.   A. Cut back salt for controlling HTN.

40.   C. The thalamus is the relaying center of the cortex.

41.   D. Assess vitals (bleeding), dyspnea, and dislodgement (ECG) after a pacemaker insertion.

42.   A. Check the ECG for V-fib/V-tach and clinical status before defibrillation.

43.   B. The blood-brain barrier protects the brain from harmful agents in the blood.

44.   C. In older adults, diminished sensory receptors due to degenerative changes lead to a reduced sense of touch, temperature, and pain.

45.   C. Explain the procedure to a patient before a cardiac cath.

46.   A. According to HIPAA, only people involved with direct patient care, insurance reimbursement, and patient management are authorized recipients of protected health information. Patients must specify in their medical records who may access their data.

47.   D. Obtain an informed consent with an immediate family member's contact number.

48.   A. Lymphedema due to lymph flow obstruction has occurred after a right-sided breast mastectomy.

49.   A. Pacemakers help maintain healthy HR.

50.   C. You will feel better after the medication.

51.   C. SBP drop > 30 mm Hg may indicate end-organ failure.

52.   A. Iron is essential for RBC production in the bone marrow.

53.   C. An HTN patient complaining of reduced exercise tolerance should exercise with restful periods.

54.   A. Stomach resection, partial or total, can deplete intrinsic factors, leading to impaired RBC production and pernicious anemia.

55.   A. Treat hypovolemia before managing the hypertensive crisis with vasoactive drugs.

56.   B. Herniation of the brain is the most critical effect of raised intracranial tension.

57.   C. The patient probably has iron deficiency anemiA. A low hemoglobin is expected in this case.

58. C. Platelet count < 150,000/µL is thrombocytopenia and can increase the risk for bleeding, demanding special consideration in nursing care.

59. C. Patients with a pacemaker should wear a MedicAlert bracelet.

60. A. Nitrates can cause dizziness and orthostatic hypotension. The patient should sit or lie down and keep the tablet under the tongue.

61. C. Thrombocytopenia causes petechiae and purpura.

62. D. Routine bedside monitoring of hemodynamic instability includes checking the vitals, urine output, capillary refill time, PP, and MAP.

63. A. Alert older patients (susceptible to orthostatic hypotension) when taking nitrates; they should change their positions slowly.

64. B. Catecholamine tests are ordered to diagnose tumors.

65. C. Unstable angina can rupture stable atherosclerotic plaque, causing thrombus.

66. B. PCI is done to open blocked coronary arteries.

67. A. Angina pain is relieved by rest or nitroglycerin, whereas MI pain is not.

68. B. Normal CVP is 1–8 mm Hg.

69. B. Suction and administer 100% oxygen.

70. A. The initiating dose of dopamine infusion is 5 mcg/kg/min.

71. C. Dopamine is the first-line drug to treat shock due to unknown causes.

72. D. Hydrochlorothiazide causes sodium and potassium loss through the kidneys. Dietary potassium foods or potassium supplements can prevent hypokalemiA.

73. A. Adequate nutrition is vital in boosting liver cell regeneration. However, severe anorexia of viral hepatitis may require careful nursing planning.

74. C. 250 IU of insulin is used to prepare insulin infusion.

75. D. The correct method to record BP is to take two or more readings at least one minute apart.

76. B. Serum bilirubin, direct and indirect, would increase in cirrhosis.

77. A. 100 mg = 0.1 gram. The nurse will give one tablet.

78. D. Fluid accumulated in the peritoneum is shunted into the venous system, releasing pressure on esophageal veins. More volume returns to the circulation, improving kidney perfusion.

79. B. A UAP can check postural changes in BP as ordered.

80. B. Dobutamine infusion is prepared in D5W.

81. C. Abstinence from alcohol is essential in alcoholic cirrhosis and can improve liver function in early cases.

82. C. A strangulated femoral hernia blocks blood supply, requiring emergency surgery.

83. C. Hypertensive emergency develops over hours or days with significantly elevated BP and evidence of acute target organ disease (cerebrovascular, cardiovascular, renal, or retinal).

84. B. Allow 30 to 45 minutes for the infusate to remain inside the rectum to expel the feces.

85. C. PID is a high risk for future infertility. The nurse should allow the patient to express her emotions, clarify her worries, and help deal with disease outcomes.

86. B. Regular insulin is used to make an infusion.

87. C. In patients with thyroid disease, palpation can release thyroid hormones into circulation, with the likelihood of causing a thyroid storm.

88. B. A normal colostomy stoma with mild to moderate edema appears bright red—a small amount of bleeding or oozing may occur on the touch.

89. D. Hypertensive crises require IV antihypertensive drugs.

90. C. A total hysterectomy leaves the ovaries intact; the patient doesn't need hormone replacement.

91. A. Insulin infusion is prepared in 250 mL of normal saline.

92. B. In confirmed pregnancy, uterine cramps with vaginal bleeding suggest spontaneous abortion.

93. B. Frequent mouth care for patients with small intestinal obstructions with an NG tube is essential.

94. A. The treatment goal is to reduce the MAP by 20% to 25% in the first hour, gradually reducing it over the next 24 hours. MAP = (SBP + 2DBP)/3. Or, MAP = 172; 25% of 172 is 129.

95. B. The QT interval is measured by estimating the R-R interval.

96. B. Ectopic pregnancy can lead to hypovolemic shock. Close monitoring of vital signs and patient condition is essential.

97. D. EBP helps clinical decision-making with excellent scientific data from patient and practitioner experiences.

98. C. Sotalol can cause QT prolongation.

99. A. The medicine has 120/5 = 24 mg/mL. Thus, the nurse will give 30/24 = 1.25 mL/dose.

100.   A. IV fluid replacement, antibiotics, NG suction, analgesics, and surgery are included in the treatment protocol.

101.   D. Endocrine system dysfunctions often cause nonspecific symptoms and diagnostic difficulties. However, goiter, exophthalmos, and the three "polys" can be considered typical.

102.   D. Diabetic foot ulcers are associated with infection and comorbidities. They are complex wounds.

103.   D. Isolating the client will not improve their condition.

104.   A. Except for buprenorphine, the rest are used for procedural sedation.

105.   B. A minimum of eight hours of overnight fasting is advisable to ensure the estimation of the fasting serum sugar level.

106.   B. The "D" of delirium mnemonic stands for dehydration.

107.   A. Reduce stimuli in a patient with an altered mental state.

108.   B. Fatigue and mental impairment, often attributed to aging, can occur in hypothyroidism.

109.   C. Tachycardia can indicate possible beta-blocker overdosing.

110.   A. There are no perfect words/interventions; be present.

111.   D. An increased serum cortisol in Cushing syndrome can cause elevated blood pressure and blood glucose.

112.   B. Mental status evaluation determines whether the patient can manage independent living.

113.   C. Exercises can prevent functional decline.

114.   A. Glycosylated hemoglobin (A1C) assesses blood glucose control during the last three months.

115. C. Each teaspoon = 5 mL. Thus, 4 tsp is 20 mL.

116. D. A *retention enema* is best for delivering medication directly to the mucosal surface of the bowel. The patient can retain the solution for an hour or more.

117. D. Oliguria is a condition of less than 400 cc of urine output in 24 hours.

118. D. She does not need a utensil cuff because there is no contracture. Meniere's Disease causes dizziness, tinnitus, and hearing loss. Thus, the shower chair, walker, and personal sound amplifier would assist this patient in being independent during her hospitalization.

119. C. Keep the pen you are using in a dry and dark place at room temperature for 28 days.

120. B. The leading cause of ESRD is diabetic nephropathy.

121. C. A low-pitched rumbling murmur signifies mitral stenosis.

122. A. IV Hypertonic glucose (50%) can cause peripheral vein phlebitis.

123. B. 25,000 mcg = 25 mg

124. A. Avoid relying on a gag reaction to decide feeding time.

125. A. Check feeding tube integrity before each shift.

Conclusion

The word "examination" is imbued with anxiety, but it should not be for you. More than a certification, nursing requires an analytical mind and an ability to think clearly and cohesively, considering all aspects of patient care, their surroundings, family, and sociocultural conditions.

The PCCN "examination" tests just that, besides your basic nursing knowledge and skills. If you have been waiting to take the exam but couldn't bring yourself to it, you may have been denying yourself the chance to fulfill your dream.

To that purpose, this guidebook has attempted to answer many queries, clear doubts, and, in the process, dispel exam-related fears. When you solve problems in addition to reviewing the material, you will ensure success.

Avoid memorizing the questions and their answers. Instead, try to understand the rationale behind the solutions. Your search will take you through basic pathophysiology, which, in turn, will strengthen your understanding. Such coordinated study practice will build your confidence and develop an intuitive ability, essential for patient care.

Knowledge makes us humble. In the nursing profession, the patient is always your focus. When you bear that in your mind, patient care becomes the best practice. You do not need to overthink.

During the PCCN test, remember there are only four options to a question. Read the question carefully and answer *what it asks*. It may not make sense to you, or you may not have experienced it, but the question demands a particular line of thinking from you, and teaching you that mindset has been the aim of this guidebook all along.

The finest way to conclude my work is for you to implement all the techniques and resources I have provided in this guide. If you like it, please consider sharing your review on Amazon. Your positive feedback encourages me to keep thinking of ways to improve the scientific method and efficiency of knowledge acquisition.

References

Al, A. M., & Manna, B. (2022, October 17). *Wound Pressure Injury Management*. National Library of Medicine; StatPearls Publishing. https://www.ncbi.nlm.nih.gov/books/NBK532897/

Alley, W. D., Schick, M. A., & Doerr, C. (2023, July 24). *Hypertensive Emergency (Nursing)*. PubMed; StatPearls Publishing. https://www.ncbi.nlm.nih.gov/books/NBK568676/

American Association of Critical Care Nurses. (n.d.-a). *Cerification Exam Policy Handbook*. https://www.aacn.org/certification/preparation-tools-and-handbooks/~/media/aacn-website/certification/get-certified/handbooks/certpolicyhndbk.pdf?la=en

American Association of Critical Care Nurses. (n.d.-b). *Certification Exam Statistics and Cut Scores - AACN*. Www.aacn.org. https://www.aacn.org/certification/preparation-tools-and-handbooks/exam-stats-and-scores

American Association of Critical Care Nurses. (n.d.-c). *Frequently Asked Questions About PCCN Certification - AACN*. Www.aacn.org. Retrieved May 27, 2024, from https://www.aacn.org/certification/get-certified/frequently-asked-questions-about-pccn-certification#:~:text=A%3A%20PCCN%20certification%20is%20a

Andrews, P. L., & Habashi, N. M. (2009). Understanding pneumonectomy. *OR Nurse, 3*(2), 32–39. https://doi.org/10.1097/01.orn.0000347325.89970.be

Bucher, L. (2016, November 17). *Nursing Management: Dysrhythmias*. Nurse Key. https://nursekey.com/nursing-management-dysrhythmias/

CDC. (n.d.). *Multiple Cause of Death Data on CDC WONDER*. Wonder.cdc.gov. https://wonder.cdc.gov/mcd.html

Conley, S. (2016). Central Line–Associated Bloodstream Infection Prevention: Standardizing Practice Focused on Evidence-Based Guidelines. *Clinical Journal of Oncology Nursing*, *20*(1), 23–26. https://doi.org/10.1188/16.cjon.23-26

Curran, A. (2022, May 13). *Pericarditis Nursing Diagnosis and Nursing Care Plan*. NurseStudy.net. https://nursestudy.net/pericarditis-nursing-diagnosis/

Diamond, M., Peniston, H.L., Sanghavi, D., Mahapatra, S., & Doerr, C. (2023) *Acute Respiratory Distress Syndrome (Nursing)*. PubMed; StatPearls Publishing. https://www.ncbi.nlm.nih.gov/books/NBK568726/#:~:text=Acute%20respiratory%20distress%20syndrome%20(ARDS)%20is%20a%20life%2Dthreatening

Douglas, M. (2017). *Hypertension Nursing Diagnosis: 6 Care Plans for Any Patient*. Prepscholar.com. https://blog.prepscholar.com/hypertension-nursing-diagnosis-care-plan

Elsevier – Clinical Skills ⊠Cardiac Monitor Set-up and Lead Placement. (2023, November 21). Elsevier.health. https://elsevier.health/en-US/preview/cardiac-monitor-set-up-and-lead-placement

Facher, L. (2023, January 17). *The addiction crisis is causing a spike in endocarditis cases. Hospitals are struggling to respond*. STAT. https://www.statnews.com/2023/01/17/addiction-spike-endocarditis-cases-hospitals/#:~:text=Among%20drug%20users%2C%20most%20endocarditis

Hashmi, M. F., Tariq, M., Cataletto, M. E., & Hoover, E. L. (2023, August 8). *Asthma (Nursing)*. PubMed; StatPearls Publishing. https://www.ncbi.nlm.nih.gov/books/NBK568760/

Kovacs, G., & Olschewski, H. (2021). The definition of pulmonary hypertension: history, practical implications and current controversies. *Breathe*, *17*(3), 210076. https://doi.org/10.1183/20734735.0076-2021

Labib, A., & Winters, R. (2021). *Complex Wound Management*. Nih.gov; StatPearls Publishing. https://www.ncbi.nlm.nih.gov/books/NBK576385/

Lloyd-Sherlock, P., Beard, J., Minicuci, N., Ebrahim, S., & Chatterji, S. (2014). Hypertension among older adults in low- and middle-income countries: prevalence, awareness and control. *International Journal of Epidemiology*, *43*(1), 116–128. https://doi.org/10.1093/ije/dyt215

Management of post-op cardiac surgery patients. (n.d.). Department of Critical Care. https://www.mcgill.ca/criticalcare/education/teaching/icu-protocols/management-post-op-cardiac-surgery-patients

MedSchool. (2018, September 20). *The ST Segment*. Medschool.co. https://medschool.co/tests/ecg-basics/the-st-segment

O'Leary, G. M. (2021). Pulmonary arterial hypertension: An overview. *Nursing 2022*, *51*(11), 37–43. https://doi.org/10.1097/01.NURSE.0000795272.64847.1b

P Knight, B. (2022, June 13). *Patient education: Cardioversion (Beyond the Basics)*. Www.uptodate.com. https://www.uptodate.com/contents/cardioversion-beyond-the-basics

Registered Nursing. (2023, December 8). *Hemodynamics: NCLEX-RN || RegisteredNursing.org*. Www.registerednursing.org. https://www.registerednursing.org/nclex/hemodynamics/

RNpedia. (2015, July 2). *Cardiomyopathy Nursing Management*. RNpedia. https://www.rnpedia.com/nursing-notes/medical-surgical-nursing-notes/cardiomyopathy/

Rodgers, J. L., Jones, J., Bolleddu, S. I., Vanthenapalli, S., Rodgers, L. E., Shah, K., Karia, K., & Panguluri, S. K. (2019). Cardiovascular Risks Associated with Gender and Aging. *Journal of Cardiovascular Development and Disease, 6*(2), 19. National Library of Medicine. https://doi.org/10.3390/jcdd6020019

Sarah. (2013, November 14). *Nursing Care Plan & Diagnosis for Heart Cath Cardiac Catheterization*. Registered Nurse RN. https://www.registerednursern.com/nursing-care-plan-diagnosis-for-heart-cath-cardiac-catheterization/

study.com. (n.d.). *AACN PCCN (Adult) Certification: Exam Review & Study Guide*.

Vera, M. (2014, February 27). *5 Hemothorax and Pneumothorax Nursing Care Plans*. Nurseslabs. https://nurseslabs.com/hemothorax-pneumothorax-nursing-care-plans/

Vera, M. (2022). *Pneumonia Nursing Care Plans: 10 Nursing Diagnosis*. Nurseslabs. https://nurseslabs.com/pneumonia-nursing-care-plans/

Wang, Y., Zhang, L., Xi, X., & Zhou, J.-X. (2021). The Association Between Etiologies and Mortality in Acute Respiratory Distress Syndrome: A Multicenter Observational Cohort Study. *Frontiers in Medicine, 8*, 739596. https://doi.org/10.3389/fmed.2021.739596

Wolf, P. A., Abbott, R. D., & Kannel, W. B. (1991). Atrial fibrillation as an independent risk factor for stroke: the Framingham Study. *Stroke, 22*(8), 983–988. https://doi.org/10.1161/01.str.22.8.983

Zippia. (2021, January 29). *Registered nurse demographics and statistics [2021]: Number of registered nurses in the US*. Www.zippia.com. https://www.zippia.com/registered-nurse-jobs/demographics/

www.ingramcontent.com/pod-product-compliance
Lightning Source LLC
Chambersburg PA
CBHW080800300326
41914CB00055B/988